THE
PELVIC
GIRDLE

THE PELVIC GIRDLE

An approach to the examination and treatment
of the lumbo-pelvic-hip region

DIANE LEE BSR MCPA COMP

Instructor/Examiner for the Orthopaedic Division of the Canadian Physiotherapy Association

Churchill Livingstone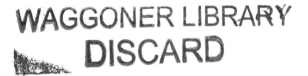

EDINBURGH LONDON MELBOURNE AND NEW YORK 1989

CHURCHILL LIVINGSTONE
Medical Division of Longman Group UK Limited

Distributed in the United States of America by Churchill
Livingstone Inc., 1560 Broadway, New York, N.Y. 10036,
and by associated companies, branches and
representatives throughout the world.

First published 1989

ISBN 0-443-03795-7

British Library Cataloguing in Publication Data
Lee, Diane
    The pelvic girdle.
    1. Man. Pelvis. Diagnosis
    I. Title
    616.7'1

Library of Congress Cataloging in Publication Data
Lee, Diane
    The pelvic girdle.
    Includes index.
    1. Pelvic girdle — Diseases. I. Title.
RC946.L44   1989   616.7'1   88–25690

Produced by Longman Singapore Publishers (Pte) Ltd.
Printed in Singapore

Preface

In 1980 it was my good fortune to have the opportunity to study with one of the leaders in manipulative therapy, Mr Cliff Fowler. Over the ensuing years I was shown how to treat people, not conditions, how to integrate academic knowledge with clinical experience and how to learn from every patient's story. At that time every story seemed to have a different stage, different players and a different plot. Through the consistent use of a basic subjective and objective examination it became apparent that there were common patterns of lumbo-pelvic-hip dysfunction. From this a logical approach to treatment has evolved.

The intent of this text is to assist the clinician in the development of a logical approach to the examination and treatment of the lumbo-pelvic-hip region based on the known anatomy, physiology and biomechanics.

Chapter 1 is a historical review of the trends of thought from Hippocrates to the present day with respect to the function and dysfunction of the pelvic girdle. Chapter 2 outlines the evolution and comparative anatomy of the pelvis followed by a description of the anatomical changes which have occurred as a result of bipedalism. This chapter is co-authored by Mr Jim Meadows whom I would like to thank both for this contribution as well as for the many hours of stimulating and thought provoking discussions.

The embryology, development and aging of the pelvic girdle is described and illustrated in Chapter 3. I would like to express my thanks to Dr J. M. Walker for providing the original photographs which illustrate the cavitation of the sacroiliac joint in the fetus, the variability in the depth of the cartilage lining the articular surfaces and the subsequent erosion and fibrous intra-articular fusion which occurs with age. The differences between the articular cartilage lining the ilium and the sacrum, as well as the changes associated with advancing age, are clearly illustrated in the original color photographs kindly provided by Dr J. D. Cassidy to whom I would like to extend my gratitude.

Chapter 4 describes and illustrates the osteology, arthrology, myology, neurology and angiology of the lumbo-pelvic-hip complex pertinent to the description and evaluation of the biomechanics of the region, which is given in Chapter 5. The theoretical section of this text is completed (Chapter 6) with a brief description of the three phases of wound repair. The clinical application of this healing process is applied in the subsequent treatment sections of Chapters 8, 9 and 10.

Chapter 7 describes and illustrates the basic subjective and objective examination of the lumbo-pelvic-hip complex. The following three chapters describe and illustrate the evaluation and treatment of the common clinical syndromes seen at the lumbosacral junction, the pelvic girdle and the hip. The

v

text is concluded with a description of the myofascial, postural and ergonomic components of therapy.

As research expands and clarifies our knowledge of the biomechanics of this region, the examination and treatment techniques can become more specific. It is hoped that this work will stimulate further research into the integrated function of the lumbar spine, the pelvic girdle and the hip and simultaneously facilitate treatment.

I woud like to extend my thanks and recognition to Mr Frank Crymble who was responsible for all the line drawings and photographs in this text. His untiring attention to detail, as well as his anatomical and artistic expertise, made working with him a pleasure. I would also like to express my appreciation and gratitude to my colleagues Mari Walsh, Jim Meadows, Cliff Fowler and Erl Pettman for their constructive reviews of this text in progress and for keeping me focused on the task at hand. Finally, to Thomas, Michael and Chelsea, for all of the hours endured, thank you.

British Columbia, 1989   D.L.

Glossary of terms

Kinematics	the study of movement
Kinetics	the study of forces
Osteo-	bone
Arthro-	joint
Myo-	muscle
Osteokinematics	the study of motion of bones regardless of the motion of the joints
Arthrokinematics	the study of motion of joints regardless of the motion of the bones
Myokinematics	the study of motion of bones produced by the contraction of the muscle
Osteokinetics	the study of forces met by the bones
Arthrokinetics	the study of forces met by the joints
Myokinetics	the study of forces met by the muscles

Contents

1

Introduction: historical review

The first medical practitioners to record interest in the pelvic girdle were the obstetricians of Hippocrates' era. Authors from Hippocrates (460–377 BC) to Vesalius (AD 1543) felt[135] that under normal conditions the sacroiliac joints were immobile; however, some practitioners felt that motion was apparent during pregnancy. This view was upheld until de Diemerbroeck (1689)[25] demonstrated that mobility of the sacroiliac joint could occur apart from the pregnant state. From the 17th century to the present date, a controversy has existed as to the classification and composition of the sacroiliac joint, the quantity, if any, of articular motion, and the specific kinematics which accompany habitual motion of the lower extremities and the trunk.

The joint has been implicated as the etiological factor in a host of symptoms including sciatica; in fact, at the turn of this century Goldthwait, Osgood[42] and Albee[4] proposed that sciatica developed from direct pressure on the lumbosacral plexus as it crossed the anterior aspect of the sacroiliac joint. This pressure was thought to be caused by 'subluxed, relaxed or diseased sacroiliac joints'.[83] Treatment consisted of manipulative reduction of the sacrum followed by immobilization for six months in spinal hyperextension via a plaster jacket. Following Mixter and Barr's[90] classic paper in 1934 on prolapsed intervertebral discs and the clinical ramifications of pressure on the lumbosacral nerve roots intra-spinally, the sacroiliac joint was no longer in the limelight and lesions of this articulation were regarded as rare.

Research over the last 50 years has revealed significant information pertaining to the kinematic and kinetic function of the pelvic girdle. It was just 75 years ago that the pubic symphysis was thought to have little importance in maintaining pelvic stability. Obstetricians at that time believed that a symphysiotomy was indicated when the 'pelvis did not properly give during labor'.[75] The obstetrician would 'make [a] high application of forceps and pull with all his brute strength and the patient [would be] rendered practically an invalid, due to injury to this joint and soft parts . . . Gradually, . . . symptoms developed . . . and the women became semi-invalids with neurasthenic symptoms, pain in the pelvis, dysmenorrhea and all the ills of women'.[4]

Despite the research which has occurred in this century, the lumbo-pelvic biomechanics which accompany movement of the lower quadrant (Ch. 5) remain controversial. That the sacroiliac joint moves is no longer the question; the specific biomechanics of the varying age groups as well as the etiological factors of dysfunction and the clinical evaluation and treatment thereof, are the subjects open to ongoing research. To facilitate this process, it is appropriate to record the current thoughts on the anatomy, biomechanics, pathophysiology and treatment of the lumbo-pelvic-hip complex. If this work stimulates further research which subsequently refutes this model, then the endeavor will have been worthwhile.

2

Evolution and comparative anatomy

In collaboration with Jim Meadows*

Author's note. The evolution of bipedalism and the consequential anatomical changes which have occurred provide some insight into the structure and function of the homo-sapien lumbo-pelvic-hip complex. For this contribution, I am indebted to Jim Meadows for his many hours of research into this subject.

INTRODUCTION

The human lumbo-pelvic-hip region, while in many respects unique in the animal world for its evolutionary adaptation to orthograde bipedalism, is based on a design originating almost half a billion years ago. The absence of fossils of typical human pelves older than five million years supports the assumption that the adaptation to bipedalism is recent. This chapter will briefly outline the steps taken in the evolutionary process which have facilitated the adoption of man's gait. Subsequently, the anatomical changes in man's structure and posture which have occurred as a consequence of bipedalism will be described.

* James Meadows MCPA MCSP COMP
Instructor for the Orthopaedic Division of the Canadian Physiotherapy Association. Education Chairman for the Orthopaedic Division of the Canadian Physiotherapy Association

EVOLUTION OF THE PELVIC GIRDLE

The pelvic girdle first appeared[29,44,92,104,111,143] as a pair of small cartilaginous elements lying in the abdomen of the primitive fish. The 'fin fold' theory maintains that lateral folds formed in the ancient fish to prevent rolling and buckling of the undulating body. Gradually, these folds fragmented secondary to their participation in propulsion and steering. From this fragmentation, two paired lateral fins were formed, the pectoral and pelvic fins. The pectoral fin was the primary propeller and was the largest and the most stable of the two. Since stability was not a functional requirement of the pelvic girdle, there was no need for axial attachment nor mutual attachment between the two sides.

With migration onto the land, the pelvic fin rapidly developed into the powerhouse of locomotion and consequently increased stability of the pelvic girdle was required. The pectoral fin (and its later development the forelimb), was relegated to the role of steering—a reversal of the original roles.

Stabilization of the pelvic girdle

The pelvic girdle has evolved towards increasing stability both at the pubic symphysis and at the sacroiliac joints. The original innominate bone contained two elements which together formed the puboischium. During the stabilization process, the puboischium enlarged and united with the opposite side via the pubo-ischial symphysis. Intra-pelvic stability was subsequently increased; however, stability between the primitive innominate bone and the axial skeleton was also required. A dorsal projection developed on the puboischium (ultimately forming the ilium) directed towards the axial skeleton.

Simultaneously, the costal element of the axial skeleton enlarged and fused with one (or more) pre-anal vertebra to form the sacrum. Then the iliac projection of the primitive innominate bone and the enlarged costal process of the primitive sacrum, which were initially united by ligaments, formed the first sacroiliac joint. Thus direct articulation between the axial and appendicular skeletons occurred. At this stage, the pelvic girdle had a full inventory of the elements that are present today in all tetrapods.

The number of vertebrae which contribute to the sacrum varies from species to species and is dependent upon the degree of stability or mobility required at the sacroiliac joint. Many amphibians and reptiles have only one or two sacral vertebrae whereas the higher mammals have five. The extreme of sacral development is found in the bird where the synsacrum includes the fusion of the sacral, lumbar and caudal thoracic vertebrae. This, together with the huge sternum, provides the stability necessary for anchoring the muscles which move the wings.

As the locomotive pattern of the vertebrates progressed from crawling to the linear-limb quadripedal and bipedal gait of the advanced mammals, the role of the ilium became more significant. The bone provided the major pelvic attachment for the limb musculature as well as the articular surface for the sacroiliac joint. This function reached its zenith in the primates and especially in the hominid ilia.

COMPARATIVE ANATOMY

The structure of man's pelvic girdle reflects the adaptation required for bipedal gait[7,34,43,64,92,103,111,117,122,131] (Fig. 2.1). The surface area of the ilia has increased whereas the length of the ischium and the pubis has decreased. The posterior muscles have lost some bulk secondary to the increased stability of the sacroiliac joint. Sufficient mobility has been maintained at this articulation for bipedalism.

Sacrum

The sacrum has increased in size thus accommodating the increased osseous attachment of the gluteus maximus muscle. The articular surface of the sacroiliac joint has also increased in size to compensate for the

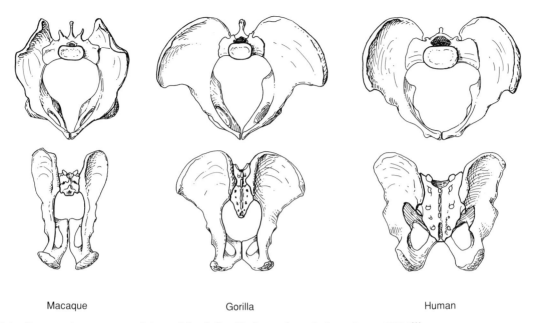

Macaque   Gorilla   Human

Fig. 2.1 Comparative anatomy of the pelvic girdle. (Redrawn from Stein & Rowe 1982.)[111]

increased compressive loading of bipedal stance. The surface itself has become more incongruous (Ch. 3) to facilitate intra-pelvic stability.

Innominate bone

The ilia have undergone dramatic changes in response to bipedalism. The bone has twisted (Fig. 2.1) such that the lateral aspect is now directed anteriorly. The gluteus medius and minimus muscles have migrated anteriorly and their function has subsequently changed. In the ape, the gluteus medius and minimus muscles are femoral extensors while in man, they act as femoral abductors (Fig. 2.2) and thus prevent a Trendelenburg bipedal gait.

In addition to the reorientation of the ilium, a fossa has developed (the iliac fossa) which increases the surface area available for the attachment of the gluteal and iliacus muscles. The reduction in extensor power caused by the anterior migration of the gluteus medius and minimus muscles is therefore compensated for. The iliac fossa also facilitates the enlargement of the iliacus muscle which plays

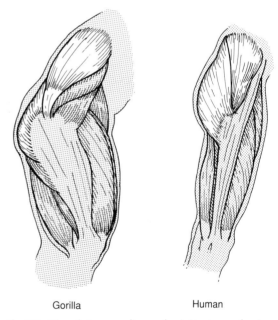

Gorilla   Human

Fig. 2.2 The gluteus medius and minimus muscles in the gorilla function as femoral extensors while in man they act as femoral abductors.

a significant role in the maintenance of man's erect posture (Ch. 5, Ch. 11).

The anatomical changes apparent in the ischium reflect the alteration in function of the hamstring muscle group (vide infra). Although these muscles have remained servile for femoral extension, constant activity is not a requirement of bipedal stance in man. Subsequently, the ischial body and tuberosity have become reduced in both length and width (Fig. 2.1). The vertical dimension of the pubic symphysis has also decreased with the evolution of efficient bipedal gait.

Acetabulum

The acetabulum has become deeper as well as reoriented in an anterolateral direction. This reorientation projects the femoral neck anteriorly and together with the angle of inclination ensures that the leg adducts at heel strike to place the foot beneath the acetabulum. The ligaments of the hip joint (Figs 4.19, 4.20) are extensive in comparison to those of the ape where they are almost non-existent.

Posture

The vertebral column of man, in comparison to other primates, differs primarily in its posture. Man's vertebral column and innominate bones have rotated posteriorly through 90° to bring the head above the feet rather than in front of them (Fig. 2.3). Although the innominate bones have rotated posteriorly, the sacrum has retained its original horizontal orientation. Consequently, the spine has become organized into a vertical column even though the orientation of the sacrum facilitated the maintenance of a horizontal row. To overcome this, the lumbar lordosis has developed. Caudally, a large lumbosacral angle developed which was compensated for by the development of a thoracic kyphosis.

In all non-human primates the lumbar spine is kyphotic. However, it is possible for a non-human primate to achieve a lumbar lordosis as was witnessed by Goodall[43] in her Gombe Stream Reserve study. One ape in this study contracted poliomyelitis as an infant which subsequently affected the function of one arm. Since the characteristic 'knuckle walk'

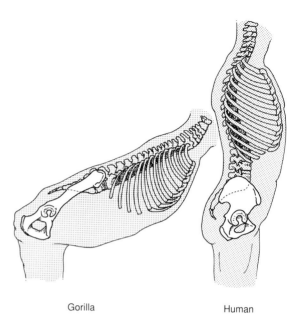

Gorilla   Human

Fig. 2.3 Posterior rotation of the vertebral column and the innominate bones has led to the development of the lumbosacral lordosis and the thoracic kyphosis.

was not possible, the animal had developed a bipedal gait for locomotion. To facilitate this, a marked lumbar lordosis had developed. However, the attachment of the gluteal muscles prevents simultaneous extension of the lumbar spine and the femur in the ape and since neither the osseous nor the myofascial structure had changed, an increase in both hip and knee flexion had to occur in order to maintain the line of gravity within the base of support.

The bipedal posture of the ape is dependent upon the massive gluteal and hamstring muscles whose major role is to stabilize the pelvic girdle and the trunk on the flexed hips. Constant activity in both muscle groups is required since the line of gravity of the bipedal ape falls considerably anterior to the coronal axis of the hip joint. Consequently, the attachments of the posterior muscles in the ape are widespread and the ischial body and tuberosity are massive. Conversely in man, the line of gravity falls slightly posterior to the coronal axis of the hip joint (Fig. 7.1) and therefore the requirements for postural balance are both reduced and reversed. The body weight is more efficiently balanced and tends to extend the pelvic girdle on the femora. To prevent this, slight recruitment of the psoas major muscle is required to maintain the optimal bipedal posture (Ch. 5). Only intermittent activity is required from the hamstring muscle group and consequently the ischial body and tuberosity have become considerably reduced in size.

SUMMARY

The human lumbo-pelvic-hip complex has developed from the primate pelvic girdle which evolved for an arboreal lifestyle. The specific osseous and myofascial adaptations for bipedalism have been relatively minor when phylogenesis is considered. The major structural changes have been in place for over three million years and appear to have resulted in the most bio-energetically efficient gait among terrestrial tetrapods. Consequently, unfinished evolutionary processes should not be regarded as the primary etiological factor in the epidemic of low back disorders. Perhaps the demands that are habitually placed on the musculoskeletal system should be incriminated instead.

3

Embryology, development and aging

EMBRYOLOGY AND DEVELOPMENT[105,131]

Development of bones

Sacrum

The sacrum derives its name from the latin word *sacer* meaning sacred. It is thought that the sacrum was the only bone to be preserved following the burning of a witch and as such must have been sacred. Fryette credits the 'ancient Phallic Worshipers [for naming] the base of the spine the Sacred Bone'.[39]

The bone is derived from the fusion of five mesodermal somites. During the 4th embryonic week, 42 to 44 pairs of somites arise from the paraxial mesoderm. Although not always consistent, the sacrum evolves from the 31st to the 35th somites each of which divides into three components—the sclerotome, myotome and dermatome (Fig. 3.1). The sclerotome multiplies and migrates both ventrally and dorsally to surround the notochord and the evolving spinal cord. Subsequently, each sclerotome divides into equal cranial and caudal components separated by a sclerotomic fissure which in the sacrum progresses to develop a rudimentary intervertebral disc composed of fibrocartilage. The adjacent sclerotomic segments then fuse to form the centrum of the sacral vertebral body. The dorsal aspect of the sclerotome which has migrated posteriorly forms the vertebral arch (the neural arch is part of this), while the ventrolateral aspect becomes the costal process (ala of the sacrum) (Fig. 3.2). This

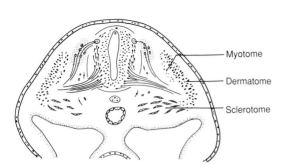

Fig. 3.1 Differentiation of the mesodermal somite into sclerotome, myotome and dermatome. (Redrawn from Warwick & Williams 1973.)[131]

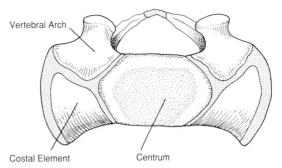

Fig. 3.2 The sclerotome of the future sacrum differentiates into three parts—the centrum, the vertebral arch and the costal element or process.

process appears only in the upper two or three sacral segments and is responsible for forming the auricular sacral surface.

Chondrification of the sacrum precedes ossification and begins during the 6th embryonic week. The primary ossification centers for the centrum and each half of the vertebral arch appear between the 10th and the 20th week, while the primary centers for the costal elements appear later, between the 6th and the 8th month.

The three components of the sacral segment (Fig. 3.2), the costal element, the vertebral arch and the centrum, remain separated by hyaline cartilage up until 2 to 5 years of age when the costal element (ala of the sacrum) unites with the vertebral arch. This unit then fuses to the centrum and to the other vertebral arch in the 8th year.

The conjoined costal element, vertebral arch and centrum of each sacral segment remain separated from those above and below

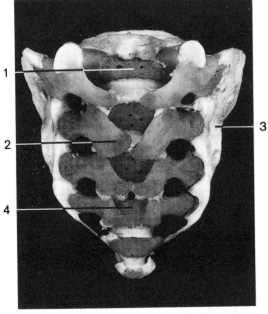

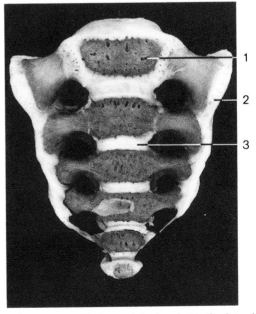

Fig. 3.3 Ossification of the sacrum. *Left*—Posterior aspect: note the centrum (1), the vertebral arch (2), the lateral epiphysis (3) and the sacral canal (4). *Right*—Anterior aspect: note the centrum (1), the lateral epiphysis (2) and the intervertebral disc (3). (Reproduced with permission from Rohen & Yokochi, Color Atlas of Anatomy. A Photographic Study of the Human Body, Published by F. K. Schattauer Verlag GmbH, Stuttgart; and Igaku-Shoin Ltd, Tokyo and New York, 1983.)

by hyaline cartilage laterally and by fibrocartilage medially (Fig. 3.3). A cartilaginous epiphysis extends the entire length of the lateral aspect of the sacrum. Fusion of the sacral segments occurs after puberty in a caudocranial direction with the simultaneous appearance of secondary ossification centers for the centrum, spinous process, transverse processes and costal elements. The adjacent margins of the sacral vertebrae ossify after the 20th year; however, the central portion of the intervertebral disc can remain unossified even after middle life.

Innominate bone

The innominate bone has a latin derivative, *in nominatus,* meaning having no name. The innominate bone appears during the 7th embryonic week as three bones, the ilium, the ischium and the pubis which are derived from a small proliferating mass of mesenchyme from the somatopleure in the developing limb bud. Three primary ossification centers appear before birth, one for the ilium above the sciatic notch during the 8th intra-uterine week, one for the ischium in the body of the bone during the 4th month and one for the pubis in the superior ramus between the 4th and 5th months. At birth, the iliac crest, the acetabular fossa and the inferior ischiopubic ramus are cartilaginous (Fig. 3.4). The latter ossifies during the 7th to 8th year. The iliac crest and the acetabular fossa develop secondary ossification centers during puberty but can remain unossified until 25 years of age.

Clinically, adolescents are frequently seen with a diagnosis of 'traumatic subluxation' of the sacroiliac joint. It is pertinent to recall the stage of development of the sacrum and the innominate bones before applying vigorous mobilization techniques to a 'bone' which is not yet a true bone.

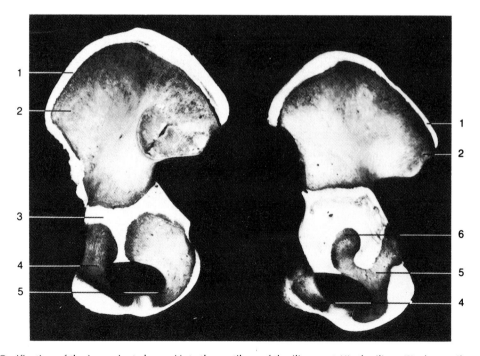

Fig. 3.4 Ossification of the innominate bone. Note the cartilage of the iliac crest (1), the ilium (2), the cartilage separating the ilium, pubis and ischium (3), the pubis (4), the ischium (5) and the acetabulum (6). (Reproduced with permission from Rohen & Yokochi, Color Atlas of Anatomy. A Photographic Study of the Human Body, Published by F. K. Schattauer Verlag GmbH, Stuttgart; and Igaku-Shoin Ltd, Tokyo and New York 1983.)

Development of joints

Sacroiliac joint

According to Bellamy[10] the development of the sacroiliac joint commences during the 8th week of intrauterine life. As in other synovial joints, a trilayer structure initially appears in the mesenchyme between the ilium and the costal element of the sacrum. Cavitation begins both peripherally and centrally by the 10th week and by the 13th week the enlarged cavities are separated by fibrous septae. These findings are not consistent with Walker's[128,129] study of 36 fetuses in which she noted that cavitation did not begin until the 32nd week (Fig. 3.5). The stage at which cavitation is complete and the fibrous bands disappear is controversial. Bellamy[10] states that the cavity is fully developed by the 8th month and that the fibrous septae soon disappear whilst Walker[128,129] notes that unlike most synovial joints which show complete cavitation by the 12th week, the sacroiliac joint remains separated by fibrous bands at birth and she questions their persistence in some joints into adulthood. Bowen[17] reports that the 10 specimens studied in this age group did not contain the fibrous septae previously noted in late fetal life. Schunke[107] was the first to describe these intra-articular bands and felt that they disappeared in the first year of life.

The synovium of the joint develops from the mesenchyme at the edges of the primordial cavity, as does the articular capsule which is thin and pliable at this stage.[17] All investigators note[17,107,129] the macroscopic and microscopic differences between the cartilage which lines the articular surfaces of the ilium and the sacrum, although the specific histological components of these surfaces remain a controversial issue today.[128]

The ilium is lined with a type of fibrocartilage which is bluer, duller and more striated than the hyaline cartilage which lines the

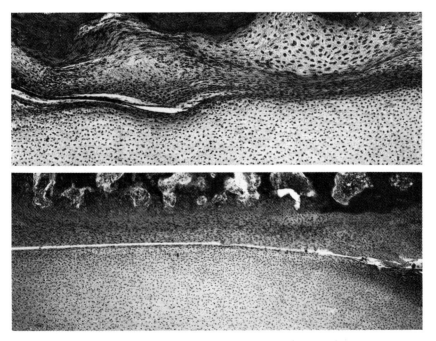

Fig. 3.5 Cavitation of the sacroiliac joint. *Top*—Sacroiliac joint of a fetus at 16 weeks of gestation. Note the proximity of the iliac bone to the joint surface, the partial cavitation of the joint and the presence of a fibrous band connecting the two surfaces. *Bottom*—Sacroiliac joint of a fetus at 34 weeks of gestation. Note that cavitation is almost complete except for a few loose fibrous bands. (Reproduced with permission from Walker 1986.)[129]

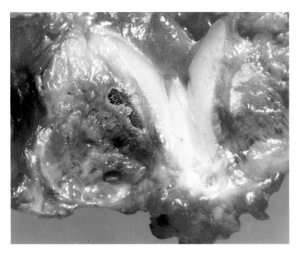

Plate 1 Sacroiliac joint of a fetus at 37 weeks of gestation. Note that the fibrocartilage lining the articular surface of the ilium is bluer than the hyaline cartilage lining the articular surface of the sacrum.

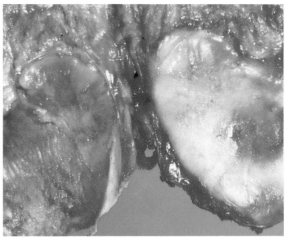

Plate 3 Sacroiliac joint of a male, 17 years of age (the sacral surface is on the right). Note the dull, rough fibrocartilage lining the articular surface of the ilium.

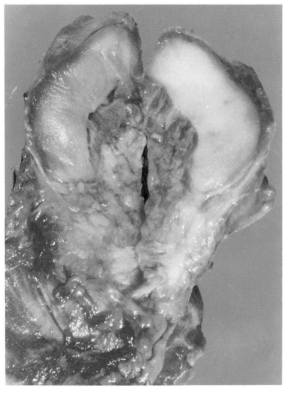

Plate 2 Sacroiliac joint of a male, 3 years of age (the sacral surface is on the right). Note the blue, dull fibrocartilage lining the articular surface of the ilium.

sacrum (Plates 1, 2). The depth of the cartilage is also different. According to Bowen,[17] the sacral hyaline cartilage is 3 to 5 times thicker than the iliac fibrocartilage. This is consistent with the findings of Schunke[107] and MacDonald,[77] although differs from the studies of Walker[129] who found that the sacral hyaline cartilage was 1.7 times thicker than the iliac fibrocartilage, although this finding may vary depending upon which aspect of the joint was being studied. All agree that the corresponding articular surfaces were smooth and flat at this stage, although Walker[128] found elevations and depressions on her full-term infants as well. Bowen[17] notes that during handling of the fetal pelves, passive articular gliding in a multitude of directions was possible, but he did not attempt a kinematic analysis.

Pubic symphysis and hip joint

Very few investigators have researched the developmental anatomy of the pubic symphysis and a reference could not be found pertaining to the anatomical changes which may occur at this articulation with advancing age.

It is beyond the scope of this text to describe the detailed embryology of the hip

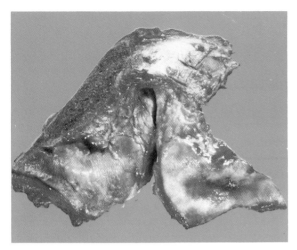

Plate 4 Sacroiliac joint of a male, 40 years of age (the sacral surface is on the right).

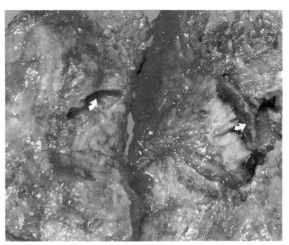

Plate 5 Sacroiliac joint of a female, 72 years of age (the sacral surface is on the left). Note the marked loss of articular cartilage on both sides of the joint as well as the presence of an accessory sacroiliac joint (arrows). (Plates 1–5 are reproduced with permission from Bowen & Cassidy 1981 and the publishers Harper and Rowe.)[17]

joint; however, several references are included for the interested reader.[108,114,125,126,127,132]

THE AGING PROCESS OF THE SACROILIAC JOINT

At birth, the pelvic girdle is far from complete developmentally. A major part of the unit is cartilaginous and the articular anatomy contributes little to intra-pelvic stability. The changes which occur within the sacroiliac joints over the next seven decades are significant to the biomechanics, assessment and treatment of the pelvic girdle with respect to the varying age groups of clinical presentation.

The first decade (0–10 years)

Bowen[17] studied seven pelves in this age group and reports that the surfaces of the sacroiliac joint remain primarily flat (Plate 2) with the major restraint to motion being provided by the very strong interosseous ligaments. The articular cartilage remains as noted prenatally.

The second and third decades (11–30 years)

The availability of cadavers for investigation in

this age group is limited; the data obtained is therefore, based on few specimens. Sashin's[106] investigation of age-related intra-articular changes is perhaps the most extensive; 42 specimens in his study belonged to this age group. Resnick's[101] study included only two specimens, MacDonald's[77] seven, Bowen's[17] seven and Walker's[129] none.

Early in the second decade the sacroiliac joint appears planar; however, by the beginning of the third decade all specimens manifest a convex ridge which runs along the entire length of the articular surface of the ilium apposed to a corresponding sacral groove.[17] The iliac fibrocartilaginous surface is duller, rougher and intermittently coated with fibrous plaques (Plate 3). The deep articular cartilage is microscopically normal, but the superficial layers are fibrillated and some crevice formation and erosion occurs by the end of the third decade. The sacral hyaline cartilage takes on a yellowish hue although macroscopic degenerative changes are not evident at this stage. The collagen content of the fibrous capsule increases, thus reducing its extensibility. Passive articular motion is limited to a posterosuperior/anteroinferior translation of the innominate bone on the sacrum.[17]

The fourth and fifth decades (31–50 years)

All investigators[17,107,128,129] agree that degeneration of the sacroiliac joint begins as early as the fourth decade. The changes occur earlier in males (fourth decade) than females (fifth decade).

The articular surfaces increase in irregularity with marked degenerative arthrosis occurring on the iliac side by the end of the fourth decade (Plate 4). Plaque formation and peripheral erosion of cartilage progress to subchondral sclerosis of bone on the iliac side. The joint space contains flaky, amorphous debris. The articular capsule thickens but still permits the translatory motion noted in the second and third decades.[17] Bony hypertrophy with some lipping of the sacral articular margins was noted in some specimens in the fifth decade.

The sixth and seventh decades (51–70 years)

At this stage (Figs 3.6, 3.7), the articular surfaces become totally irregular with deep erosions occasionally exposing the subchondral bone. Peripheral osteophytes enlarge and often bridge the anterior margin and inferior lip of the joint.[17,101] Fibrous interconnections between the articular surfaces are commonplace; however, 'when stressed, all specimens maintained some degree of mobility, although this was restricted when compared with the younger specimens'.[17]

The eighth decade (over 70 years)

Intra-articular fibrous connections are more often the rule with some periarticular osteophytosis present (Plate 5, Fig. 3.8). Cartilaginous erosion and plaque formation is extensive and universal, filling the joint space with debris. Consequently, the joint space is markedly reduced. Intra-articular bony ankylosis is rarely reported and usually thought to be associated with ankylosing spondylitis (Fig. 3.9). Schunke[107] reports that the average age of the specimens with bony ankylosis is considerably less than those without fusion, confirming a probable pathological cause.

In Walker's study, 15 adult cadavers between 49 and 84 years of age were investigated for age-related changes. 'Changes observed in adult specimens were similar to those of previous reports, but from examination of the entire joint, this report emphasizes the inherent variability of the sacroiliac joint, both within and between joints, at any of the ages studied'.[129]

SUMMARY

That the sacroiliac joint degenerates with time is not unique to this articulation. The clinical

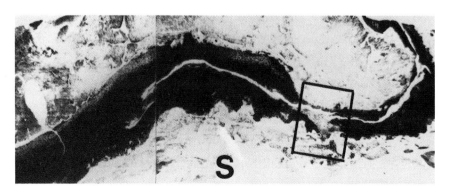

Fig. 3.6 Sacroiliac joint of a male, 60 years of age. Note the variability in the depth of both the sacral (S) and the iliac cartilage at different sites. (Reproduced with permission from Walker 1986.)[129]

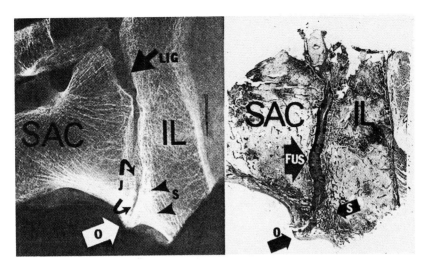

Fig. 3.7 *Left*—This radiograph of a coronal section through the sacroiliac joint of a cadaver over 70 years of age illustrates narrowing of the joint space (J), sclerosis of the bone (S) and osteophyte formation (O) secondary to the degenerative process. Note the space for the interosseous ligament (LIG). *Right*—This photomicrograph reveals the thickened trabeculae in the sclerotic region (S) and an area of fibrous intra-articular fusion (FUS). (Reproduced with permission from Resnick et al 1975, and the publishers J. B. Lippincott.)[101]

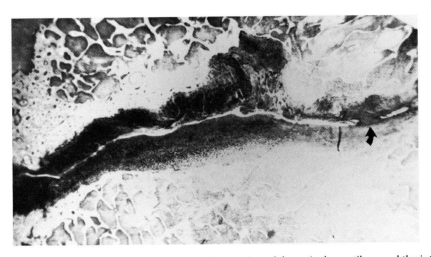

Fig. 3.8 Sacroiliac joint of a female, 81 years of age. Note the erosion of the articular cartilage and the intra-articular fibrous connection (arrow). (Reproduced with permission from Walker 1986.)[129]

significance of the effects of degeneration on articular mobility is a controversial issue. There is an ongoing debate between researchers and clinicians as to the absence of scientific verification for the various examination procedures, diagnostic interpretations and subsequent treatment techniques applied to the pelvic girdle. Unfortunately, cadaver dissections and static biomechanical analysis can not replicate living anatomy nor duplicate habitual movement of the lower extremity either in weight-bearing or in non-weight-bearing. In the light of current scientific data, the presence or absence of sacroiliac joint mobility and its significance to the patient's presenting complaints are best judged by accurate, objective, clinical evaluation. In the absence of bony intra-articular ankylosis, the

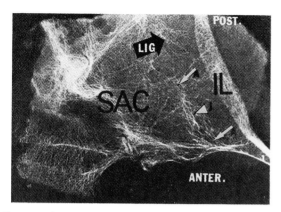

Fig. 3.9 This radiograph of a transverse section through the sacroiliac joint (J) illustrates the intra-articular ankylosis (A) of ankylosing spondylitis. Note the ossification of the interossetous ligament (LIG). (Reproduced with permission from Resnick et al 1975, and the publishers J. B. Lippincott.)[101]

clinical impression is that age does not preclude motion—the individual's ontogeny may just be slightly behind his time.

4

Anatomy

HISTORY

The earliest record of anatomical data pertaining to the pelvic girdle is credited to Bernhard Siegfried Albinus (1697–1770) and William Hunter (1718–1783).[75] These anatomists were the first to demonstrate that the sacroiliac joint was a true synovial joint, a finding confirmed by Meckel in 1816. Von Luschka, in 1854, was the first to classify the joint as diarthrodial. Further anatomical studies conducted by Albee[4] in 1909 on 50 postmortem specimens confirmed that the joint was lined with a synovial membrane and contained by a well-formed articular capsule. His findings were confirmed by Brooke[20] in 1924. It wasn't until 1938 that the variations in the articular cartilage lining the iliac surface were noted.[107] In 1957, Solonen[110] conducted a comprehensive study of the osteology and arthrology of the pelvic girdle, from which some findings will be reported later.

The pelvic girdle as a unit supports the abdomen as well as provides a dynamic link between the vertebral column and the lower limbs. It is a closed osteoarticular ring composed of six or seven bones which include the two innominate bones, the sacrum, the one or two bones which together form the coccyx and the two femora, as well as six or seven joints which include the two sacroiliac, the sacrococcygeal, often an intercoccygeal, the pubic symphysis and the two hip joints.

OSTEOLOGY (the bones)

Sacrum

> Little wonder that the ancient Phallic Worshipers named the base of the spine the Sacred Bone. It is the seat of the transverse center of gravity, the keystone of the pelvis, the foundation of the spine. It is closely associated with our greatest abilities and disabilities, with our greatest romances and tragedies, our greatest pleasure and pains.[39]

The sacrum is a large triangular bone situated at the base of the spine wedged between the two innominate bones. It is formed by the fusion of five sacral vertebrae (see Fig. 3.3), and the vertebral equivalents are easily recognized. The sacrum is highly variable both between individuals and between the left and right sides of the same bone. In spite of this, certain anatomical features are consistent and only those which are essential to the description and evaluation of sacral function (Ch. 5 and Ch. 7) will be described here.

The cranial aspect of the first sacral vertebra (Fig. 4.1), the sacral base, consists of the vertebral body anteriorly (the anterior projecting edge being the sacral promontory) and the vertebral arch posteriorly. Laterally, the transverse processes of the first sacral vertebra are fused with the costal elements (see Fig. 3.2) to form the alae of the sacrum.

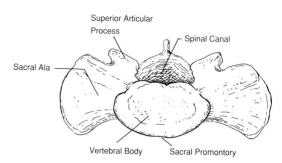

Fig. 4.1 The cranial aspect of the first sacral vertebra—the sacral base.

Variations have been noted[48] in the height of the sacral alae as well as the body of the S1 vertebra. The orientation of the superior articular processes of the S1 vertebra is also variable (vide infra).

The posterior surface of the sacrum (Fig. 4.2) is convex in both the coronal and the transverse planes. The spinous processes of the S1 to S4 vertebrae are fused in the midline to form the median sacral crest. Lateral to the median sacral crest, the intermediate sacral crest is formed by the fused laminae of the S1 to S5 vertebrae. The laminae and inferior articular processes of the S5 (and occasionally the S4) vertebra remain unfused in the midline. They project caudally to form the sacral cornua, and together with the posterior

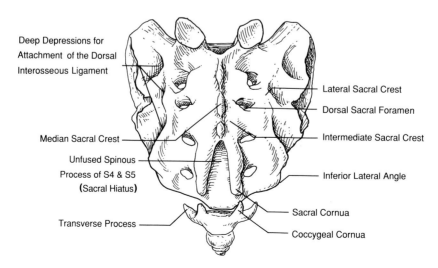

Fig. 4.2 The posterior aspect of the sacrum and coccyx.

aspect of the vertebral body of the S5 vertebra form the sacral hiatus. The lateral sacral crest represents the fused transverse processes of the S1 to S5 vertebrae. Between this crest and the intermediate sacral crest lie the dorsal sacral foramina which transmit the dorsal sacral ramus of each sacral spinal nerve. There are three deep depressions in the lateral sacral crest at the levels of the S1, S2 and S3 vertebrae. These depressions contain the strong attachments of the interosseous sacroiliac ligament (Figs 4.2, 4.13).

The lateral sacral crest fuses with the costal element to form the lateral aspect of the sacrum (Fig. 4.3). Superiorly the lateral aspect of the sacrum is wide, while inferiorly the anteroposterior dimension narrows to a thin border which curves medially to join the S5 vertebral body. This angle is called the inferior lateral angle of the sacrum (Figs 4.2, 4.4). The L-shaped auricular surface of the sacrum is contained entirely by the costal elements of the first three sacral segments.

The short arm of the L-shaped surface (Fig. 4.3) has an inferosuperior axis and is contained within the first sacral segment. The long arm lies in an anteroposterior plane within the second and third sacral segments. The contours of the articular surface are reported[60,110,134,135] to be highly variable depending upon the age of the individual studied (see Ch. 3). Investigators have reported[60] the presence of a curved furrow

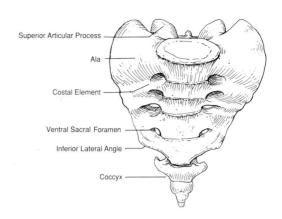

Fig. 4.4 The anterior aspect of the sacrum and coccyx.

bordered by two longitudinal crests corresponding to a convex longitudinal crest on the articular surface of the ilium. However, Solonen in his study of 30 skeletons concluded that there were 'numerous depressions, elevations and other irregularities . . . In no case was there a distinct ridge—furrow or eminence depression formation. On the contrary, the impression was gained that great irregularity prevails in respect to the surface formations'.[110] His study, however, did not consider the age-related changes which may have been present in his specimens.

The anterior surface of the sacrum (Fig. 4.4) is concave in both the coronal and the transverse planes. In the midline, four interbody ridges represent the sclerotomic fissures which are not always completely fused. Lateral to the fused vertebral bodies are four ventral sacral foramina which transmit the ventral ramus of each sacral spinal nerve as well as the segmental ventral sacral artery. The costal elements project laterally from the middle of each vertebral body between the ventral sacral foramina and fuse with those above and below as well as with the transverse processes posteriorly to form the lateral aspect of the sacrum.

The orientation of the articular surface of the sacrum in both the coronal and the transverse planes has been studied by Solonen[110] and a summary of his findings is presented in Table 4.1. These observations represent the common findings but variations were noted.

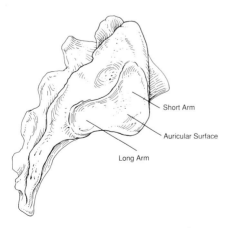

Fig. 4.3 The lateral aspect of the sacrum.

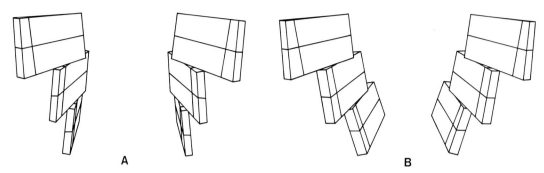

Fig. 4.5 Steriometric drawings of two pelves studied by Solonen[110] illustrating the variation found in the orientation of the sacral articular surface. (Redrawn from Solonen 1957.)[110]

Table 4.1 Orientation of the articular surface of the sacrum in the coronal and transverse planes as described by Solonen[110] and as shown graphically in Figure 4.5

Coronal plane	Fig. 4.5:
90% of the specimens examined narrowed inferiorly at S1	A and B
85% of the specimens examined narrowed inferiorly at S2	B
80% of the specimens examined narrowed superiorly at S3	A
Transverse plane	
S1 and S2 narrow posteriorly	
S3 narrows anteriorly	

The steriometric drawings of two pelves studied by Solonen are illustrated in Figure 4.5.

Fryette[39] examined 23 sacra and subsequently classified the bone into three types—A, B, and C (Figs 4.6, 4.7, 4.8). This classification is dependent upon the orientation of the sacral articular surface in the coronal plane which he found correlated with the orientation of the superior articular processes of the S1 vertebra. The Type A sacrum narrows inferiorly at S1 and S2 and superiorly at S3. The orientation of the superior articular processes in this group is in the coronal plane. The Type B sacrum narrows superiorly at S1 and the orientation of the superior articular processes in this group is in the

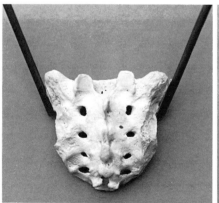

Fig. 4.6

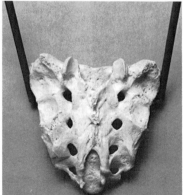

Fig. 4.7

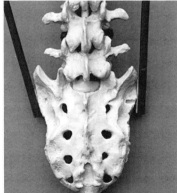

Fig. 4.8

Figs 4.6 to 4.8 Sacrum types A, B and C.

sagittal plane. The Type C sacrum narrows inferiorly at S1 on one side (Type A) and superiorly at S1 on the other (Type B). The orientation of the superior articular processes is in the coronal plane on the Type A side and in the sagittal plane on the Type B.

In conclusion, there is a high incidence of variability in the plane of the sacroiliac joint both in the coronal and the transverse planes as well as in the shape of the articulating surfaces. Grieve has noted that 'Each joint exhibits at least two planes slightly angulated to one another and often three—their disposition and area are not always similar when sides are compared in the same individual'.[49] As clinicians, we are never relieved of the necessity for accurate clinical evaluation given the anatomical uncertainty of the individual being assessed.

Coccyx

The coccyx (Figs 4.2, 4.4) is represented by four fused coccygeal segments although the first is commonly separate. The bone is roughly triangular, the base bears an oval facet which articulates with the inferior aspect of the S5 vertebral body. The first coccygeal segment contains two rudimentary transverse processes as well as two coccygeal cornua which project superiorly to articulate with the sacral cornua.

Innominate bone

There are three parts to the innominate bone, the ilium, the ischium and the pubis which in the adult are fused to form one bone, the innominate (Figs 4.9, 4.10 and see Fig. 3.4). Only the anatomical features pertinent to the description and evaluation of function of the innominate bone will be described here.

Ilium

The ilium is a fan-like structure forming the superior aspect of the innominate bone and contributes to the superior portion of the acetabulum. The iliac crest is convex in the sagittal plane and sinusoidal in the transverse plane such that the anterior portion is concave medially while the posterior portion is convex medially. The curve reversal occurs in the same coronal plane as the short arm of the L-shaped articular surface. At either end of the iliac crest a bony projection will be found, the anterior superior iliac spine (ASIS) anteriorly and the posterior superior iliac spine (PSIS)

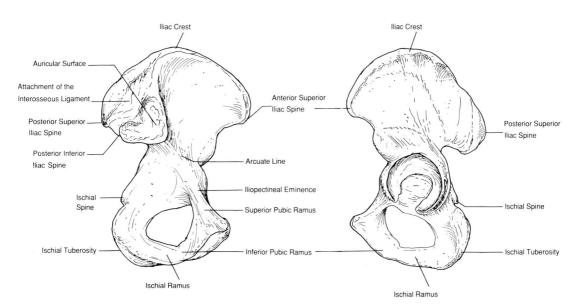

Figs 4.9 and 4.10 The medial and lateral aspects of the innominate bone.

posteriorly. Inferior to the PSIS, the ilium curves irregularly to end at the posterior inferior iliac spine (PIIS). The sacroiliac joint can be palpated directly at this point. It is often the site of an accessory sacroiliac joint.[110,120]

Several anatomical points are worthy of note on the medial aspect of the ilium. The auricular surface lies on the posterosuperior aspect of the medial surface. Like the sacrum, the articular surface is L-shaped with the axis of the short arm in the inferosuperior plane, while the long arm has an anteroposterior axis. A variety of elevations, depressions, ridges and furrows have been reported, possibly consistent with age-related changes (see Ch. 3). Although the elevations and depressions are found on both the iliac and sacral articular surfaces, they are not a mirror image of one another.[128] Superior to the articular surface, the medial aspect of the ilium is very rough and affords attachment to the strong interosseous sacroiliac ligament which has been noted[82] to remain intact when the sacrum and the innominate bone are forced apart in cadavers. For the most part, the sacroiliac joint cannot be palpated given the depth of the articulation and this point should be noted when studying the anatomy here.

Anteriorly, the arcuate line of the ilium appears at the angle between the short and the long arms of the auricular surface and projects anteroinferiorly to reach the iliopectineal eminence, a point at which the ilium and the pubis unite. This line between the sacroiliac joint and the iliopectineal eminence represents a line of force transmission from the vertebral column to the lower limb and is reinforced by subperiosteal trabeculae (see Fig. 5.24).[60]

Pubis

The inferomedial aspect of the innominate bone is formed by the pubis which articulates with the pubis of the opposite side via the pubic symphysis. It joins the ilium superiorly via the superior pubic ramus which constitutes the anterior one-fifth of the acetabulum.

Inferiorly, the inferior pubic ramus projects posterolaterally to join the ischium on the medial aspect of the obturator foramen. The lateral surface of the pubis is directed towards the lower limb and affords attachment for many of the medial muscles of the thigh. The pubic tubercle is located at the lateral aspect of the pubic crest approximately 1 cm lateral to the midsymphyseal line.

Ischium

The inferolateral one-third of the innominate bone is formed by the ischium. The upper part of the body of the ischium forms the floor of the acetabulum as well as the posterior two-fifths of the articular surface of the hip joint. From the lower part of the body, the ischial ramus projects anteromedially to join the inferior ramus of the pubis. The ischial tuberosity is a roughened area on the posterior and inferior aspect of the ischial body and is the site of strong muscular and ligamentous attachments. Superior to the tuberosity, the ischial spine projects medially. This process is also the site of ligamentous and muscular attachments (see Figs 4.12, 4.14).

Acetabulum

The acetabulum (see Figs 4.10, 4.18) is formed from the fusion of the three bones which make up the innominate bone (see Fig. 3.4). It is roughly the shape of a hemisphere and projects in an anterolateral and inferior direction. The lunate surface represents the articular portion of the acetabulum while the non-articular portion constitutes the floor, or the acetabular fossa. This fossa is continuous with the acetabular notch located between the two ends of the lunate surface.

Femora

Clinically, it is important to note that the angle of inclination of the femoral neck to the shaft of the femur, as well as the angle of anteversion between the femoral neck and the coronal plane, are highly variable. This variability will be reflected in both the pattern and the range of motion available at the hip joint.[60]

ARTHROLOGY (the joints)

Sacroiliac joint

The sacroiliac joint (Fig. 4.11) is classified as a synovial joint or diarthrosis.[17] Albinus and Hunter[17] were the first to note the presence of a synovial membrane within the joint. Koelcher,[17] in 1850, identified synovial fluid within the joint on dissection.

The shape, as well as the articular cartilage, have been previously described (see Ch. 3). To summarize, the sacral surface is covered with hyaline cartilage while the iliac surface is covered with a type of fibrocartilage (see Plates 1–4).[128] The depth of the articular cartilage differs both within the same articular surface and on apposing sides (see Fig. 3.6). Most investigators report[17,77,110] a ratio of 1:3 between the iliac and sacral surfaces.

The joint capsule is composed of two layers, an external fibrous layer which contains abundant fibroblasts, blood vessels and collagen fibers and an inner synovial layer.[17] The chronological changes in the articular capsule have been described (Ch. 3). Anteriorly the capsule is clearly distinguished from the overlying ventral sacroiliac ligament, while posteriorly the fibers of the capsule and the deep interosseous ligament are intimately blended. In-

feriorly, the capsule blends with the periosteum of the contiguous sacral and innominate bones.

Like other synovial joints, the sacroiliac joint capsule is supported by overlying ligaments, some of which are the strongest in the body. They include the:
1. ventral sacroiliac ligament
2. interosseous sacroiliac ligament
3. dorsal sacroiliac ligament
4. sacrotuberous ligament
5. sacrospinous ligament
6. iliolumbar ligament.

Ventral sacroiliac ligament

The ventral sacroiliac ligament (Fig. 4.12) is the weakest of the group and is little more than a thickening of the anterior and inferior parts of the joint capsule.[17,131] Clinically, when the sacroiliac joint is hypermobile (see Ch. 9), this ligament is invariably attenuated and often a source of pain. The ligament can be palpated anteriorly at Baer's point (see Ch. 7). When it is responsible for the patient's complaints, the pain can be reproduced or magnified by palpation as well as by stressing this structure.

Interosseous sacroiliac ligament

The interosseous sacroiliac ligament is the strongest of the group and completely fills the space between the lateral sacral crest and the

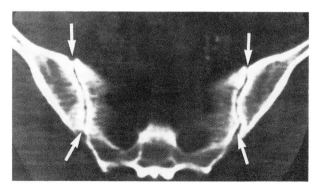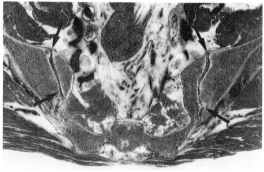

Fig. 4.11 A computed tomography scan (left) with a photograph of the corresponding anatomical section (right) through the synovial portion of a cadaveric sacroiliac joint (arrows). (Reproduced with permission from Lawson et al 1982 and the publishers Raven Press.)[68]

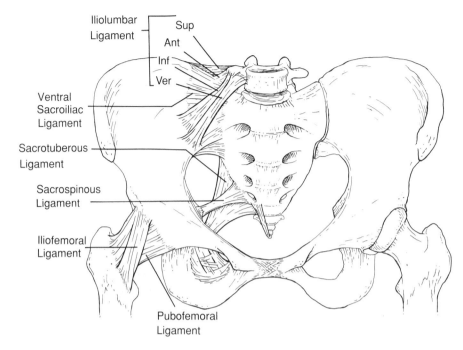

Fig. 4.12 The ligaments of the pelvic girdle viewed from the anterior aspect.

iliac tuberosity (Fig. 4.13 and see Fig. 3.7). The fibers are multidirectional and can be divided into a deep and superficial group. The deep layer attaches medially to three fossae on the lateral sacral surface (see Fig. 4.2) and laterally to the adjacent iliac tuberosity. The superficial layer of this ligament is a fibrous sheet which attaches to the lateral sacral crest at S1 and S2 and to the medial aspect of the iliac crest. This structure is the primary barrier to direct

palpation of the sacroiliac joint in its superior part and its density makes intra-articular injections extremely difficult. The strength of this ligament is greater than that of the bones to which it attaches and clinically it has yet to be shown to be attenuated.[17,82]

Dorsal sacroiliac ligament

The dorsal sacroiliac ligament attaches medi-

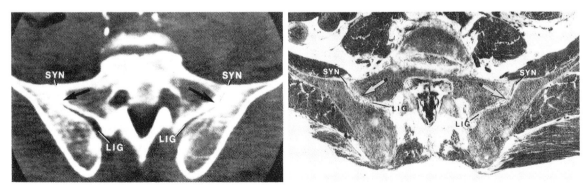

Fig. 4.13 A computed tomography scan (left) with a photograph of the corresponding anatomical section (right) through the sacroiliac joint. Note the depth of the synovial portion (SYN) of the joint and the interosseous ligament (LIG). (Reproduced with permission from Lawson et al 1982 and the publishers Raven Press.)[68]

ally to the entire length of both the intermediate and the lateral sacral crests and laterally to the posterior superior iliac spine and the inner lip of the iliac crest. As such, it contains fibers which run transversely, obliquely and vertically. It lies posterior to the interosseous ligament and is separated from it by the emerging dorsal branches of the sacral spinal nerves and blood vessels. The inferior fibers from the S3 and S4 vertebrae blend laterally with the sacrotuberous ligament and medially with the posterior layer of the thoracolumbar fascia.

This ligament thus provides a direct anatomical link between the extensors of the hip joint and the supporting fascia of the lumbar spine via the sacrotuberous ligament. The structure ideally suits the functional requirements of habitual motion (see Ch. 5).

The skin overlying the ligament is a frequent area of pain in patients with lumbosacral and pelvic girdle dysfunction. Tenderness on palpation of the dorsal sacroiliac ligament does not necessarily incriminate this tissue given the nature of pain referral (see macroscopic articular neurology, p. 35) both from the lumbar spine and the sacroiliac joint.

Sacrotuberous ligament

Phylogenetically, the sacrotuberous ligament (Figs 4.12, 4.14; and see Fig. 6.1) represents the tendinous insertion of the biceps femoris muscle in lower vertebrates.[131] In man, this ligament still receives some fibers from the biceps femoris muscle. It attaches medially to the posterior superior iliac spine, the transverse tubercles of the S3, S4 and S5 vertebrae and to the lateral margin of the lower sacrum and coccyx. Its fibers run in an inferior, lateral and anterior direction to converge into a thick band which attaches to the medial margin of the ischial tuberosity. The ligament is pierced by the perforating cutaneous nerve (S2, S3) which subsequently winds around the inferior border of the gluteus maximus muscle to supply the skin covering the medial and inferior part of the buttock, perhaps a source of paraesthesia when entrapped.

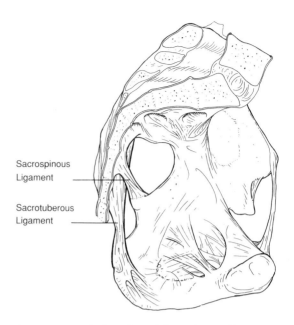

Fig. 4.14 A sagittal section of the pelvic girdle illustrating the anchoring effect of the sacrotuberous ligament on the sacral base.

This ligament is vital to the kinetic function of the pelvic girdle (see Ch. 5). The palpation of its integrity is an essential component of the pelvic girdle evaluation (see Ch. 7).

Sacrospinous ligament

The sacrospinous ligament (Figs 4.12, 4.14; and see Fig. 6.1) attaches medially to the lower, lateral aspect of the sacrum and the coccyx. Laterally, the apex of this triangular ligament attaches to the ischial spine of the innominate bone. It is closely connected to the coccygeus muscle from which it may represent a degenerated part.[131] Clinically, this ligament may be responsible for the secondary coccygodynia experienced by patients with dysfunction of the innominate bone.

Iliolumbar ligament

In a recent study,[73] the iliolumbar ligament (Figs 4.12, 4.15) was examined both macroscopically and histologically in 33 specimens ranging in age from the first to the ninth

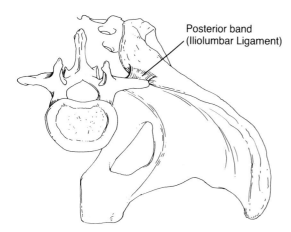

Posterior band
(Iliolumbar Ligament)

Fig. 4.15 A transverse section of the lumbosacral junction illustrating the attachment of the posterior band of the iliolumbar ligament.

decade. Macroscopically, two bands of the ligament were noted, both arising from the tip of the transverse process of the L5 vertebra. The anterior band inserts onto the anterior margin of the iliac crest while the posterior band inserts onto the posterior margin of the iliac crest. The quadratus lumborum muscle arises from, and between, these two bands. Histological analysis of the varying age groups revealed that up until the third decade the ligament is entirely muscular and can not be differentiated from the quadratus lumborum muscle. 'By the end of the second decade, the ligaments were entirely collagenous and clearly demarcated from the rest of the quadratus lumborum muscle'.[73] After the fifth decade, all of the muscle fibers had been replaced by ligamentous tissue.

> Our study has shown that the iliolumbar ligament does not exist at birth, but develops gradually in the first decade and attains full differentiation only in the second decade. The total absence of collagen fibers in the neonatal specimens and their subsequent appearance within normal muscle fibers suggests that the iliolumbar ligament is formed by metaplasia of some fibers of the quadratus lumborum muscle as a response to stresses created at the lumbosacral junction when the erect posture is assumed.[73]

Bogduk[16] describes five bands of the iliolumbar ligament—the anterior, the superior, the posterior, the inferior and the vertical. The anterior band attaches to the anteroinferior aspect of the entire length of the transverse process of the L5 vertebra. It blends with the superior band anterior to the quadratus lumborum muscle to attach to the anterior margin of the iliac crest. The superior band arises from the tip of the transverse process of the L5 vertebra. Laterally, the band divides to envelope the quadratus lumborum muscle before inserting onto the iliac crest. The posterior band also arises from the tip of the transverse process of the L5 vertebra. Laterally, it inserts onto the iliac tuberosity posteroinferiorly to the superior band. The inferior band arises both from the body and the inferior border of the transverse process of the L5 vertebra. Inferiorly, the fibers cross the ventral sacroiliac ligament obliquely to attach to the iliac fossa. The vertical band arises from the anteroinferior border of the transverse process of the L5 vertebra. These fibers descend vertically to attach to the posterior aspect of the arcuate line.

Both authors[16,73] speculate that these ligaments are responsible for maintaining the stability of the lumbosacral junction both in the coronal and the sagittal planes.

Sacrococcygeal joint

The sacrococcygeal joint is classified as a symphysis. The sacrum and the coccyx are joined via a fibrocartilaginous disc developed from the embryonic sclerotomic fissure, although occasionally the joint is synovial.[131] The supporting ligaments include the:
1. ventral sacrococcygeal ligament
2. dorsal sacrococcygeal ligament
3. lateral sacrococcygeal ligament.

The ventral sacrococcygeal ligament represents the continuation of the anterior longitudinal ligament of the vertebral column. The dorsal sacrococcygeal ligament has two layers. The deep layer attaches to the posterior aspect of the body of the S5 vertebra and the coccyx (analogous to the posterior longitudinal ligament) whereas the superficial layer bridges the margins of the sacral hiatus and the posterior aspect of the coccyx, thus completing the sacral canal (see Fig. 4.2). Laterally, the intercornual ligaments, or the lateral sacrococcygeal ligaments, connect the sacral and coccygeal cornua.

Intercoccygeal joint

The intercoccygeal joint is classified as a symphysis in the young since the first two segments are separated via a fibrocartilaginous disc. With time, the joint usually ossifies; however, it occasionally remains synovial.

Pubic symphysis

The presence of a fibrocartilaginous disc (Fig. 4.16a), as well as the absence of synovial tissue and fluid, qualifies this articulation to be classified as a symphysis. The osseous surfaces are covered by a thin layer of hyaline cartilage; however, they are separated by the fibrocartilaginous disc. The posterosuperior aspect of the disc often contains a cavity which is not seen before the age of 10 years.[131] This is a non-synovial cavity and may represent a chronological degenerative change. The supporting ligaments of this articulation (Figs 4.16a, b, c) include the:

1. superior pubic ligament
2. inferior arcuate ligament
3. posterior pubic ligament
4. anterior pubic ligament.

The superior pubic ligament is a thick fibrous band which runs transversely between

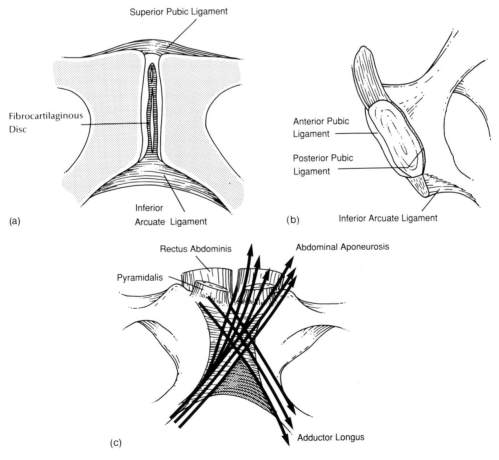

Fig. 4.16 The pubic symphysis. (a) A coronal section. (b) A sagittal section through the fibrocartilaginous disc. (c) The anterior aspect. (Redrawn from Kapandji 1974.)[61]

the pubic tubercles of the pubic bones. In-feriorly, the arcuate ligament blends with the fibrocartilaginous disc to attach to the inferior pubic rami bilaterally. The posterior pubic ligament (Fig. 4.16b) is membranous and blends with the adjacent periosteum while the anterior ligament of the pubic symphysis is very thick and contains both transverse and oblique fibers.[61] It receives fibers from the aponeurotic expansion of the abdominal musculature as well as the adductor longus muscle which decussates across the joint (Fig. 4.16c).

In health, the pubic symphysis is very stable; contrary to the obstetrical opinion at the turn of this century, it is now known[142] that the stability of this articulation is vital to both the kinetic and kinematic function of the pelvic girdle (see Ch. 5).

Hip joint

The hip joint (Fig. 4.17) is classified as a synovial joint of an unmodified ovoid shape.[76] The head of the femur forms roughly two-thirds of a sphere, and except for a small fovea it is covered by hyaline cartilage which decreases in depth toward the periphery of the surface. The acetabulum has been described (see osteology). The lunate surface of the

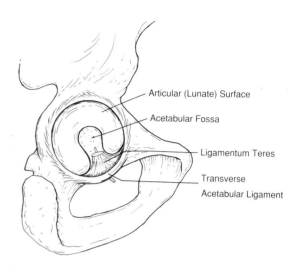

Fig. 4.18 The acetabulum.

acetabulum (Fig. 4.18) is lined with hyaline cartilage while the non-articular portion, the acetabular fossa, is filled with loose areolar tissue and covered with synovium. The acetabulum is deepened by a fibrocartilaginous labrum which on cross-section is triangular in shape (Fig. 4.17). The base of the labrum attaches to the rim of the acetabulum except inferiorly where it is deficient at the acetabular notch, which is bridged by the transverse acetabular ligament. The apex of the labrum is lined with articular cartilage and lies inside the hip joint as a free border; the capsule of the joint attaches to the labrum at its peripheral base, thus creating a circular recess.

The articular capsule encloses the joint and most of the femoral neck. Medially, it attaches to the base of the acetabular labrum and extends 5 to 6 cm beyond this point onto the innominate bone. Inferiorly, the medial attachment is to the transverse acetabular ligament. Laterally, the capsule inserts onto the femur anteriorly along the entire extent of the trochanteric line, posteriorly to the femoral neck above the trochanteric crest, superiorly to the base of the femoral neck and inferiorly to the femoral neck above the lesser trochanter. The superficial bands of the capsular fibers are predominantly longitudinal while the deep bands are circular forming the zona orbicularis (Fig. 4.17) which has few, if

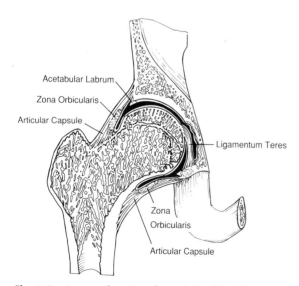

Fig. 4.17 A coronal section through the hip joint.

any, osseous connections. The zona orbicularis divides the synovial cavity into a medial and a lateral recess. The ligaments which are intimately blended with, and support, the capsule include the:
1. iliofemoral ligament
2. pubofemoral ligament
3. ischiofemoral ligament.

There are two intra-articular ligaments, the ligamentum teres and the transverse acetabular ligament.

Iliofemoral ligament

The iliofemoral ligament (Figs 4.12, 4.19, 4.20) is extremely strong and reinforces the anterior aspect of the hip joint. It is triangular in shape and attaches to the anterior inferior iliac spine at its apex. Inferolaterally, it diverges into two bands, the lateral iliotrochanteric band which inserts onto the superior aspect of the trochanteric line and the medial inferior band which inserts onto the inferior aspect of the trochanteric line. Together, these two bands form an inverted Y, the center of which is filled with weaker ligamentous tissue.

Pubofemoral ligament

The pubofemoral ligament (Figs 4.12, 4.19)

attaches medially to the iliopectineal eminence and the superior pubic ramus as well as to the obturator crest and membrane. Laterally, it attaches to the anterior surface of the trochanteric line. The capsule of the hip joint is unsupported by any ligament between the pubofemoral ligament and the inferior band of the iliofemoral ligament; however, the tendon of the psoas major muscle crosses the joint at this point contributing to its dynamic support. A bursa is located here between the tendon of the psoas muscle and the capsule and occasionally will communicate directly with the synovial cavity of the hip joint.

Ischiofemoral ligament

The ischiofemoral ligament (Fig. 4.20) arises medially from the posterior aspect of the acetabulum and its labrum. Laterally, the fibers spiral superoanteriorly over the back of the femoral neck to insert anterior to the trochanteric fossa deep to the iliofemoral ligament. Some fibers from this ligament also run transversely to blend with those forming the zona orbicularis.

Ligamentum teres

The ligamentum teres (Figs 4.17, 4.18) attaches

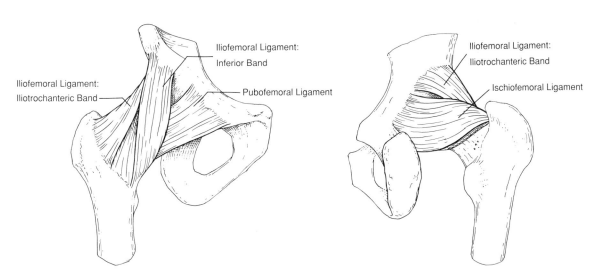

Fig. 4.19 The ligaments of the anterior aspect of the hip joint.

Fig. 4.20 The ligaments of the posterior aspect of the hip joint.

laterally to the anterosuperior part of the fovea of the femoral head and medially via three bands to either end of the lunate surface of the acetabulum inferiorly and to the upper border of the transverse acetabular ligament.

Transverse acetabular ligament

This ligament is a continuation of the acetabular labrum inferiorly and converts the acetabular notch into a foramen through which the intra-articular vessels pass to supply the head of the femur (Fig. 4.18).

In addition to the ligamentous support, the hip joint is dynamically stabilized by numerous muscles including the iliacus, rectus femoris, pectineus, gluteus minimus, piriformis, obturator externus, obturator internus, superior and inferior gemellus muscles as well as the fascia lata of the thigh, all of which partially insert into the articular capsule.

MYOLOGY (the muscles)

There are 35 muscles which attach directly to the sacrum and/or innominate bone and function with the ligaments and fascia to produce synchronous motion of the trunk and the lower extremities. They also provide the dynamic stability necessary for both upper and lower quadrant motion. They include the following:
 1. latissimus dorsi
 2. external oblique
 3. internal oblique
 4. transverse abdominis
 5. rectus abdominis
 6. pyramidalis
 7. gluteus medius
 8. gluteus minimus
 9. gluteus maximus
10. piriformis
11. superior gemellus
12. inferior gemellus
13. obturator internus
14. obturator externus
15. semimembranosus
16. semitendinosus
17. biceps femoris
18. quadratus femoris
19. adductor brevis
20. adductor longus
21. adductor magnus
22. pectineus
23. gracilus
24. rectus femoris
25. sartorius
26. tensor fascia lata
27. erector spinae
28. quadratus lumborum
29. iliacus
30. psoas minor
31. levator ani
32. sphincter urethrae
33. superficial transverse perineal and ischiocavernosus
34. coccygeus
35. multifidus.

Although 'Classic myology, with its emphasis on origins and insertions, often fails to convey the dynamism of an active contracting structure exerting a force between its two fixed ends',[34] some anatomical review is required to facilitate the subsequent discussion of biomechanics and clinical syndromes. The reader should refer to a good anatomy text for detail on the muscles listed but not described below.

Of the 35 muscles which attach to the innominate bone, six attach to the sacrum. Note that all of the muscles which attach to the sacrum, arise from, or insert onto, the innominate bone as well.

Multifidus

The following myological description is from the work of Bogduk[15,16] who has done extensive research on the anatomy of the vertebral column.[11-16] The results of his work are significantly different from reputed anatomy texts[131] and offer possible explanations for some of the clinical syndromes seen in the lumbar spine (see Ch. 8).

The deepest fibers of the multifidus muscle in the lumbar spine (the laminar fibers) arise from the posteroinferior aspect of the lamina and insert *two* levels below onto the mammillary process. The remainder of the muscle arises medially from the spinous process, blending laterally with the laminar fibers. Inferiorly, the fascicles insert *three* levels below such that those arising from the L1 vertebra insert onto the mammillary processes of the L4, L5 and S1 vertebrae as well as the medial aspect of the iliac crest. Inferiorly, the fibers from the spinous process of the L2 vertebra insert onto the mammillary processes of the L5 and S1 vertebrae and the PSIS of the innominate bone. The fibers from the spinous process of the L3 vertebra insert onto the S1 articular process, the superolateral aspect (costal element) of the S1 and S2 segments and the iliac crest. The fibers from the spinous process of the L4 vertebra insert onto the lateral sacral crest and the area of bone between this crest and the dorsal sacral foramina while those from the L5 vertebra insert onto the intermediate sacral crest inferiorly to S3.

The fascicles are innervated by the medial branch of the dorsal ramus such that all of the fascicles which arise from the same spinous process are innervated by the same nerve regardless of the inferior extent of their insertion.[12]

Due to the anatomical attachments, this muscle is capable of influencing the motion of bones which do not directly articulate. As shall become evident later, the osseous, articular, myofascial and neurological components of the lumbar spine, pelvic girdle and hip joints are interdependent both anatomically and physiologically. Dysfunction rarely implicates only one part of the system; this facilitates treatment but complicates a specific 'diagnosis' as well as research.

Erector spinae

Lumbar longissimus

This muscle (Fig. 4.21) arises from five muscle laminae, the deepest of which is from the L5 vertebra overlapped by those from L4, then L3, then L2 and finally L1.[15,16] Medially, these

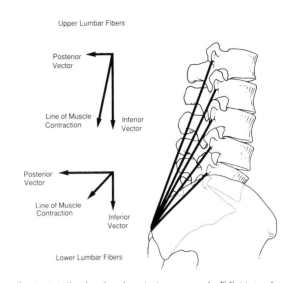

Fig. 4.21 The lumbar longissimus muscle.[15,16] Note the relative posterior orientation of the fibers from the L5 vertebra as opposed to the inferior orientation of the fibers from the L1 vertebra. The force vectors which occur as a result of contraction of the muscle are depicted on the left. The lower lumbar fibers have a greater posterior 'pull' than the upper lumbar fibers which have a greater inferior 'pull'. (Redrawn from Bogduk 1986.)[15]

laminae arise from the segmental transverse and accessory processes. Laterally, the fibers from the L1 to L4 vertebrae insert via a common tendon into the medial aspect of the lumbar intermuscular aponeurosis which attaches inferiorly to the PSIS of the innominate bone. The fibers from the L5 vertebra pass more posteriorly than inferiorly in comparison to the fibers from the L1 vertebra which pass more inferiorly than posteriorly to insert onto the medial aspect of the PSIS. Consequently, the lower fibers act unilaterally as segmental rotators and bilaterally as posterior translators. Clinically, the lower fibers may be responsible for producing the lumbar kyphosis, or rotoscoliosis, seen in patients with an acute L5–S1 joint dysfunction. A myofascial etiology could explain the rapid restoration of the lumbar lordosis following treatment with neuromuscular inhibition techniques (i.e active mobilization, functional, counterstrain).[50]

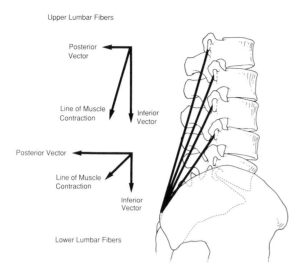

Upper Lumbar Fibers

Posterior Vector

Line of Muscle Contraction

Inferior Vector

Posterior Vector

Line of Muscle Contraction

Inferior Vector

Lower Lumbar Fibers

Fig. 4.22 The lumbar iliocostalis muscle.[15,16] Note the relative posterior orientation of the lower fibers and the omission of attachment to the L5 vertebra. The force vectors which occur as a result of contraction of the muscle are depicted on the left. The lower lumbar fibers have a greater posterior 'pull' than the upper lumbar fibers which have a greater inferior 'pull'. (Redrawn from Bogduk 1986.)[15]

Lumbar iliocostalis

This muscle (Fig. 4.22) arises as four overlapping laminae from the tips of the transverse processes of the L1 to L4 vertebrae. Inferiorly, the muscle inserts onto the PSIS and the superior aspect of the iliac crest 3 to 5 cm lateral to the PSIS. The inferior laminae from the L4 vertebra have a more posterior orientation than the superior fibers from the L1 vertebra. Bogduk[11,15,16] notes that this muscle is a more effective rotator than the lumbar longissimus muscle since its attachment is further lateral on the transverse process, and hence has a longer lever arm.

Thoracic longissimus and thoracic iliocostalis

According to Bogduk[15,16] these two muscles are not confined to the thorax but span several segments to gain attachment both to the PSIS of the innominate bone and to the aponeurosis of the erector spinae muscle which covers the lumbar longissimus muscle before attaching to the posteroinferior aspect of the sacrum. Consequently, these muscles are also capable of influencing the motion of bones which do not directly articulate.

Quadratus lumborum

A pertinent point to note here is the attachment of this muscle to the superior and anterior bands of the iliolumbar ligament.[16,73] This muscle may contribute to the dynamic stability of the lumbosacral junction by increasing the tension of the iliolumbar ligament.

Gluteus maximus

This muscle attaches extensively to the pelvic girdle via the:
1. posterior gluteal line of the innominate bone
2. aponeurosis of erector spinae muscle
3. dorsum of the lower lateral sacrum
4. coccyx
5. sacrotuberous ligament
6. fascia covering the gluteus medius muscle.
In man, less than a half of this muscle attaches directly to the gluteal tuberosity of the femur while the remainder inserts into the iliotibial tract of the fascia lata.[34] Its function will be discussed in detail under myokinematics and myokinetics.

Piriformis

The piriformis muscle arises from the anterior aspect of the S2, S3 and S4 segments of the sacrum as well as the capsule of the sacroiliac joint, the anterior aspect of the PIIS of the ilium, and often the upper part of the sacrotuberous ligament. Its exit from the pelvis is through the greater sciatic foramen (see Fig. 6.1) and it attaches to the greater trochanter of the femur.

It has been proposed[79,88,119] that altered function of this muscle may be responsible for restricting sacroiliac joint motion and/or producing local pain. Entrapment neuropathies of the sciatic nerve as it passes through and/or beneath the piriformis muscle can occur. Trigger points located in this muscle as well as the gluteus medius, longissimus and multifidus muscles have been reported[119] to refer pain to the sacroiliac joint.

With regard to the 'piriformis syndrome',[66,79,80,85,93] Grieve notes:

> Because muscle tenderness of itself has not engendered elsewhere in the body a host of muscle syndromes like trapezius syndrome, deltoid syndrome, sacrospinalis syndrome, gluteal syndrome, gastrocnemius syndrome and so on, it may appear somewhat indiscriminative to attach such importance to the name of a tender muscle as to propose a clinical entity on the basis of what is almost certainly a 2° [secondary] consequence.[48]

Rectus abdominis

A key myological point to note concerning this muscle is the inferior attachment to the pubic symphysis. The aponeurotic expansions of this muscle, along with those of the transversus abdominis, internal oblique, pyramidalis and adductor longus muscles, interdigitate anterior to the symphysis to form a dense network of fibers and thus contribute to the stability of this articulation (see Fig. 4.16c).[61,131]

Pyramidalis

This triangular muscle is located anterior to the inferior aspect of the rectus abdominis muscle and is enclosed within its sheath. The base attaches to the os pubis as well as to the symphysis while the apex blends with the linea alba midway between the umbilicus and the pubis. This muscle is innervated by the subcostal nerve which is the ventral ramus of the T12 spinal nerve. Clinically, superoinferior asymmetry of the pubic symphysis can be effectively treated by restoring the function of the T12–L1 spinal segment. Perhaps the pyramidalis muscle, via altered neurophysiology from the T12–L1 spinal segment, is responsible for maintaining the clinically observed distortion of the pubic symphysis. Reflecting back to the arthrology of this articulation, it is difficult to envisage an articular etiology for this asymmetry.

Levator ani

This muscle, together with its fellow on the opposite side, forms a greater part of the pelvic floor. Anteriorly, it attaches to the body of the pubis and posteriorly, to the medial aspect of the ischial spine. Between these two points it attaches to the obturator fascia. In the midline posteriorly, fibers attach to the last two coccygeal segments. From this point, a median fibrous raphe extends anteriorly from the apex of the coccyx to the anorectal flexure.

In the midline anteriorly decussating muscular fibers cross the prostate gland in the male and the vagina in the female, while posteriorly the muscular fibers cross, and some blend with, the rectum.

Though rarely reported spontaneously, a common subjective complaint in patients with pelvic girdle distortion is pain during sexual intercourse and/or defecation. This muscle could conceivably be responsible if the pelvic girdle asymmetry was sufficient to alter the muscle's resting length and subsequently the anal and vaginal apertures.

Iliacus

The iliacus muscle arises from the iliac fossa, the ventral sacroiliac ligament and the inferior fibers of the iliolumbar ligament,[15,16] as well as the lateral part (costal element) of the sacrum. Distally, its fibers converge to merge with the lateral aspect of the tendon of the psoas muscle while some go on to insert directly onto the lesser trochanter of the femur. As it crosses the hip joint, some fibers attach to the upper part of the capsule.

Psoas minor

This muscle is absent in 40% of the population and when present arises from the sides of the bodies of the T12 and L1 vertebrae as well as the intervertebral disc.[131] Distally, it inserts onto the iliopectineal eminence of the innominate bone. It is supplied by the ventral ramus of the L1 spinal nerve. This muscle may be responsible for the 'snapping hip' or deep clunk occasionally found on active hip flexion in one-legged standing. This symptom is difficult to treat (possibly because the exact etiology is not known) and attention should be directed to the thoracolumbar junction due to the muscle's nerve supply.

Psoas major

Although this muscle does not directly attach to either the innominate bone or the sacrum, its influence on the biomechanics of the region is significant and it would be remiss not to include its description. The muscle attaches to the anteroinferior border of the transverse processes of the L1 to L5 vertebrae as well as to the intervertebral discs and adjacent vertebral bodies. Medially, it blends with the tendinous arch which spans the waist of each vertebral body beneath which pass the segmental nerves and blood vessels.

Inferiorly, the muscle fibers converge into a tendon which receives the iliacus muscle medially before crossing the anterior aspect of the hip joint between the iliofemoral and pubofemoral ligaments. Inferiorly, the tendon inserts onto the lesser trochanter of the femur. The tendon is separated from the capsule of the hip joint by the iliopsoas bursa. The muscle is innervated via the ventral rami of the L1 and L2 spinal nerves, and hence the neurophysiological connection to the thoracolumbar junction.

The fascia

The fascia of the lower extremity envelopes the muscles and via its extensive attachments to the pelvic girdle can influence its function and subsequently become symptomatic in dysfunction. The fascia encircles the pelvic girdle by attaching to the sacrum, coccyx, iliac crest, inguinal ligament, superior pubic ramus, inferior pubic ramus, ischial ramus, ischial tuberosity and sacrotuberous ligament. Superiorly, it blends with the thoracolumbar and abdominal fascia of the trunk. From the iliac crest, the fascia descends over the gluteus medius muscle before splitting to envelope the gluteus maximus muscle. The two bands meet at the lower border of this muscle and facilitate its insertion into the iliotibial tract which represents a lateral thickening of the fascia.

The iliotibial tract attaches inferiorly to the condyles of the femur and the tibia, and to the head of the fibula blending with the crural fascia and aponeurotic extensions of the quadriceps muscle. The fascia is continuous in the thigh with two intermuscular septa which attach to the linea aspera.

The tensor fascia lata muscle inserts into the iliotibial tract anterior to the attachment of the gluteus maximus muscle. This muscle is also enveloped by two layers of the fascia. The superficial layer reaches the iliac crest lateral to the muscle while the deep layer blends medially with the capsule of the hip joint.

NEUROLOGY (the nerves)

The understanding of the neurology of the lumbo-pelvic-hip complex is essential since rehabilitation involves the restoration of optimal neurological function. The muscular control of the lumbo-pelvic-hip complex in posture and locomotion is directly dependent upon both the central and peripheral nervous systems. Janda notes that 'It is almost impossible clinically to differentiate the primary changes in muscle from their secondary reaction due to an altered or impaired central nervous regulation, as the quality of muscle function depends directly on the central nervous system activity'.[56]

Wyke[140,141] has shown that articular neurology has both direct and reflex influences on muscle tone locally and globally as well as contributing to perceptual experiences of postural sensation and kinesthesis. Altered afferent input from the articular mechanoreceptors can have profound influences on both static and dynamic pelvic girdle function.

Macroscopic articular neurology

Rudinger (1857) is reported[110] to be the first to describe the macroscopic innervation of the sacroiliac joint. It is a subject which does not appear to have been investigated extensively—especially histologically.

The most extensive study of the macroscopic innervation of the sacroiliac joint was done in 1957 by Solonen[110] who examined 18 joints in nine cadavers and found that posteriorly all of the joints were innervated from branches of the posterior rami of the S1 and S2 spinal nerves. More recently (1985), Bradlay[18] reported that the dorsal sacroiliac ligaments, and presumably the joint, receive supply from the lateral divisions of the dorsal rami of the L5, S1, S2 and S3 spinal nerves. The lateral branches of the L5, S1 and S2 dorsal rami form a plexus between the dorsal sacroiliac and interosseous ligaments from which the joint is innervated.

Anteriorly, Solonen[110] found that the articular innervation was not always consistent nor necessarily symmetrical. Of the 18 specimens examined, all of the joints were innervated by branches from the ventral rami of the L5 spinal nerve, 17 from L4, 11 from S1, 4 from S2, 1 from L3 and 15 received innervation from the superior gluteal nerve. The clinical significance of this variation may be reflected in the wide variety of pain patterns reported by patients with sacroiliac joint dysfunction.

The hip joint is innervated by branches from the obturator nerve (L2, L3, L4), the nerve to quadratus femoris (L2, L3, L4) and the superior gluteal nerve (L5, S1).[50,54] As well, the joint receives branches from the nerves which supply the muscles crossing the joint. The hip joint is principally derived from the L3 segment of mesoderm with contributions from L2 to S1; hence the potential for a variety of patterns of pain referral.

Contrary to Wyke's[140,141] reports, Bogduk[12,15,16] states that the outer one-third of the lumbar intervertebral disc is innervated posteriorly by the sinuvertebral nerve and laterally by the ventral rami and gray rami communicantes of the spinal nerve. Nocicep-

tors have been located here, thus the anatomical potential for primary disc pain. The zygapophysial joints of the L5 and S1 vertebrae are innervated via the medial branch of the dorsal ramus of the L4, L5 and S1 spinal nerves.

Microscopic articular neurology

A reference could not be found which directly reported on the presence or absence of Type I or II mechanoreceptors in the capsule of the sacroiliac joint. Although Wyke reports that 'these corpuscles have been observed in all the joints we have examined without exception',[140] he does not note if the sacroiliac joint was specifically examined. The hip joint capsule has been studied by Dee[26] and a brief review of his findings is presented below.

Type I mechanoreceptors are found in all regions of the superficial capsule of the hip joint, being the most dense in the inferior, anterior and posterior aspects. A few of these receptors are found in the femoral attachment of the ligamentum teres.[140] Some of the receptors emit a continuous low frequency discharge whilst others respond to capsular tension by increasing their frequency of discharge. Together these receptors report on both the static and dynamic joint position, thus contributing to kinesthetic sensation with information on the direction, degree and velocity of joint motion. They also respond to intra-articular pressure changes. They are a low threshold, slowly adapting receptor stimulated by an increase in tissue tension, whether intra-articular or extra-articular in origin. Given the number of muscles which attach to the hip joint capsule, articular motion is not necessary to fire these receptors.[140] Alterations in the resting tone of the muscles attaching to the hip joint capsule will significantly alter the afferent input received centrally from these receptors.

Type II mechanoreceptors are sparsely located in the deeper layers of the hip joint capsule and in the acetabular fat pad.[26] These receptors have a low threshold but they adapt rapidly and do not emit a resting discharge. They are stimulated by mechanical tension which stresses the tissue in which they are located and fire predominantly at the beginning and the end of joint motion; hence they are dynamic receptors.

Type III mechanoreceptors are located both in the intra-capsular and extra-capsular ligaments. There is an abundance of these receptors in the ligamentum teres.[118] They are high threshold receptors and therefore require an excessive amount of stress to activate a discharge. They adapt very slowly and have a powerful reflex inhibitory effect on some, or all, of the ipsilateral muscles which cross the joint.[26] When the Type III receptors in the ligamentum teres are discharged, all of the muscles about the hip joint are inhibited with the exception of the glutei which are facilitated.

Type IV receptors are located at the end of three-dimensional lattice-like plexuses throughout the joint capsule, periosteum, fat pads, and adventitial sheaths of the blood vessels. Free nerve endings with Type IV receptors are found in all of the intra-capsular and extra-capsular ligaments. Both systems respond to extremes of mechanical deformation and/or chemical irritation (potassium, ions, lactic acid, polypeptide kinins, 5-hydroxy-tryptamine, acetylcholine, noradrenalin, prostaglandins, histamine) and are high-threshold, non-adapting receptors. These receptors contribute to the perception of pain (nociception); however, the afferent input can be significantly altered both peripherally and centrally.

According to Wyke[140] the central effects of articular mechanoreceptor activity are threefold:

1. Reflex

   Depolarization of the afferent fibers from the Type I and Type II mechanoreceptors reaches the fusimotor neurons polysynaptically, thus contributing to the gamma-feedback loop from the muscle spindle both at rest and during joint motion. 'By this means the articular mechanoreceptors exert reciprocally coordinated reflexogenic influences on muscle tone and on the excitability of stretch reflexes in all the striated muscles'.[141] When this capsular reflex is activated the discharging receptors facilitate the muscles antagonistic to the occurring movement. As previously mentioned, when the Type III mechanoreceptors are discharged, the reflex effect is projected polysynaptically to the alpha-motoneurons and results in local muscular inhibition. When the Type IV receptors are discharged, the alpha-motoneurone pool is affected, thus distorting the normal, coordinated, mechanoreceptor reflex system and producing abnormalities in posture and movement.

2. Perceptual

   Afferent input from the Type I mechanoreceptors travels polysynaptically via the posterior and dorsal spinal columns to reach the paracentral and parietal regions of the cerebral cortex, thus contributing significantly, though not solely, to both postural and kinesthetic awareness. 'The observation that capsulectomy of the hip joint performed in the course of hip replacement surgery does not result in total loss of postural sensation at the hip, leaves no doubt that while joint capsule mechanoreceptors contribute to awareness of static joint position, they are not the sole source of perceptual experience, and other recent studies suggest that their contribution in this regard is supplementary to and coordinated with that provided by the inputs from cutaneous and myotatic [muscle spindle] mechanoreceptors!'[141]

3. Pain suppression

   'No matter where it is felt in the body, and no matter from what cause, pain—which is the commonest of all clinical symptoms encountered in medical practice—represents a disturbance of neurological function'.[48] Unlike taste, touch or smell, pain is not a primary neurological sensation but rather a complex neurological phenomenon influenced by patterns of activity in specific afferent systems as well as by past and present experiences.

Impulses subserving pain are not transmitted centrally by small diameter fibers only. The entire spectrum of afferent fibers may be stimulated by peripheral noxious stimuli, depending upon the intensity of the stimulus. The experience of pain depends upon mechanisms of convergence, summation and modulation both peripherally in the spinal cord and centrally in the brain stem and cortex.

The theory of peripheral modulation, or spinal gating, was originally proposed by Melzak and Wall.[84] Briefly, the gate-control mechanism is dependent upon large fiber activity (mechanoreceptor) which presynaptically inhibits the transmission of impulses from the small fiber nociceptors at the substantia gelatinosa. Thus 'by rhythmic movement of the body, or a body part, and by cutaneous contact and soft tissue compression, i.e. stroking, holding and by rhythmic manual or mechanical mobilization techniques, the large diameter (6–12 microns and 13–17 microns) mechanoreceptors are stimulated'[48] and subsequently modulate the transmission of nociceptor activity.

Centrally, the perception of pain can be influenced by psychological factors including past experience, anxiety and culture, and drugs such as caffeine, alcohol and barbiturates, all of which increase the experience of pain.

The study of pain is a text in itself and all practitioners dealing with it should be familiar with the complex nature of this neurological dysfunction.

Table 4.2 The peripheral nerves and their spinal root derivatives which innervate the muscles of the pelvic girdle

Muscle	Peripheral nerve	Roots
Abdominals	Ventral rami	T12, L1
Pyramidalis	Subcostal nerve	T12
Gluteus medius	Superior gluteal	L5, S1
Gluteus minimus	Superior gluteal	L5, S1
Gluteus maximus	Inferior gluteal	L5, S1, S2
Piriformis	Ventral rami	L5, S1, S2
Superior gemellus	Nerve to obturator internus	L5, S1
Inferior gemelllus	Nerve to quadratus femoris	L5, S1
Obturator externus	Obturator	L3, L4
Obturator internus	Nerve to obturator internus	L5, S1
Quadratus femoris	Nerve to quadratus femoris	L5, S1
Semimembranosus	Tibial	L5, S1, S2
Semitendinosus	Tibial	L5, S1, S2
Biceps femoris	Tibial, common peroneal	L5, S1, S2
Adductor brevis	Obturator	L2, L3, L4
Adductor longus	Obturator	L2, L3, L4
Adductor magnus	Obturator, tibial	L2, L3, L4
Pectineus	Femoral, accessory obturator	L2, L3
Gracilus	Obturator	L2, L3
Rectus femoris	Femoral	L2, L3, L4
Sartorius	Femoral	L2, L3
Tensor fascia lata	Superior gluteal	L4, L5
Erector spinae	Lateral and intermediate branches of the segmental dorsal rami	
Quadratus lumborum	Ventral rami	T12–L3(4)
Iliacus	Femoral	L2, L3, L4
Psoas minor	Ventral rami	L1
Levator ani	Inferior rectal, pudendal	S4
Sphincter urethra	Perineal branch pudendal	S2, S3, S4
Coccygeus	Ventral rami	S4, S5
Multifidus	Medial branch of segmental dorsal ramus	
Psoas major	Ventral rami	L1, L2, L3

Muscular neurology

The peripheral nerves and their spinal root derivatives which innervate the muscles of the pelvic girdle are found in Table 4.2.

ANGIOLOGY (the blood supply)

The hip joint is supplied by the obturator, the medial and lateral femoral circumflex and the superior and inferior gluteal arteries and veins.[23,49,54,109] The acetabular fossa, its contents as well as the head of the femur, receive supply from the acetabular branch of the obturator and medial femoral circumflex vessels via the ligamentum teres (see Fig. 4.18). The vascular anatomy is inconsistent and rarely sufficient to sustain the viability of the head of the femur following interruption of other sources of supply. 'Experimental findings[6] point to a connection between aching pain, elevation of intraosseous pressure and impaired [venous] drainage of spongiosa. Rhythmic mobilizations of this articulation are extremely effective in relieving persistent aches associated with osteoarthritis. Together with the effects of mechanoreceptor discharge during these techniques perhaps improved circulation plays a role in pain suppression'.[49]

The nutrient arteries and veins for the sacrum arise from the lateral and median sacral system. The lateral sacral vessels arise from the posterior trunk of the internal iliac and descend over the anterolateral aspect of the sacrum. The two longitudinal arteries give off anterior central branches which course medially to anastamose with the median sacral artery. The anterior central branches send feeder vessels into the centrum of the sacrum. At the level of the ventral sacral foramina, spinal branches supply the cauda equina as well as the contents of the sacral canal. The foraminal branch, after passing through the dorsal sacral foramina, supplies the posterior aspect of the medial and intermediate sacral crests as well as the posterior musculature. Venous drainage is via vessels which accompany the arteries and subsequently drain into the common iliac system.

The nutrient supply for the innominate bone is derived from the iliac branches of the obturator and iliolumbar vessels as well as the superior gluteal vessels.[131] A reference could not be found which described the blood supply to the sacroiliac joint.

5

Biomechanics of the lumbo-pelvic-hip complex

The primary function of the lower quadrant of the body is to locomote as well as to provide a stable base from which the upper quadrant can operate. Together, the trunk and the lower extremities have the potential for multidimensional movement with a minimum of energy expenditure. Neuromusculoskeletal harmony is essential for optimal lumbo-pelvic-hip function. Meisenbach in 1911 stated that 'When the trunk is moved to one side quickly there are direct opposing forces of the lumbar and spinal muscles against the pelvic and leg muscles. Normally these work in harmony and are resisted by the strong pelvic ligaments and fascia to a certain extent. If the harmony of these muscles is disturbed from some cause or another, or if the ligamentous support is weakened, other points of fixation must necessarily yield'.[83]

So how do the bones, the joints and the muscles achieve this harmonious action? Before discussing the integrated biomechanics of the lumbo-pelvic-hip region, a description of the terminology used in this text is required.

DEFINITION OF TERMINOLOGY

The terms kinematics (the study of movement) and kinetics (the study of forces) come from the science of kinesiology, the study of biomechanics (Table 5.1). The prefixes osteo-, arthro- and myo- are Greek derivatives

39

Table 5.1 Definition of biomechanical terminology[48,131]

Term	Definition
Kinematics	The study of motion of particles and rigid bodies without consideration of the forces involved
Kinetics	The study of the effects of forces on the motion of materials
Osteo-	Bone
Arthro-	Joint
Myo-	Muscle

meaning bone, joint and muscle respectively.

Osteokinematics refers to the study of motion of bones regardless of the motion of the joints. 'All bones move at joints. But the kinematics of a bone does not require any inquiry into the kinematics of the joint at which the bone moves. The bone is considered simply as an object moving in space, an object that can be studied without opening the joint'.[76] These motions are named according to the axis about which they occur (see Figs 5.1, 5.27).

Flexion/extension occurs when one or more bones rotate(s) about a coronal axis. Abduction/adduction occurs when one or more appendicular (peripheral) bones rotate(s) about a sagittal axis. Sideflexion occurs when an axial bone (skull, vertebral column) rotates about a sagittal axis. Medial/lateral rotation occurs when one or more appendicular (peripheral) bones rotate(s) about a vertical or longitudinal axis. Axial rotation occurs when an axial bone (skull, vertebral column) rotates about a vertical or longitudinal axis. The bones can also translate along the same axes resulting in posteroanterior, mediolateral and vertical (distraction–compression) translation.

Arthrokinematics refers to the study of motion of joints regardless of the motion of the bones. 'Intra-articular kinematics or arthrokinematics has to do with the movement of one articular surface upon another . . . Articular surfaces can spin and/or slide upon each other'.[76] These motions are referred to as pure spins and pure and impure swings. A pure spin occurs when the only motion of a point on the articular surface is a rotation around the mechanical axis of the bone. A pure swing occurs when the only motion of a point on the articular surface is a slide along the shortest possible line (the chord) between two points. An impure swing occurs when a point on the articular surface slides along any other curved line (an arc) between two points such that an element of spin also occurs.

Myokinematics refers to the study of motion of bones produced by the contraction of the muscle. 'Myokinematics has to do with the way in which the structure and arrangement of a set of muscle fibers determines the amount of angular motion associated with its full contraction, and so the range of movement it can help to occur'.[76]

Osteokinetics, arthrokinetics and myokinetics refer to the study of forces met by the bones, joints and muscles during static and dynamic function.

LUMBOSACRAL JUNCTION—KINEMATICS

The kinematic analysis of the lumbosacral junction pertains to the quantitative and qualitative study of the motion of the L5 vertebra (and its joints) relative to the sacrum during physiological movement. Newton's second law states that the motion of an object is directly proportional to the applied force and occurs in the direction of the straight line in which the force acts. Translation occurs when a single net force causes all points of the object to move in the same direction over the same distance.[16] Rotation occurs when two unaligned and opposite forces cause the object to move around a stationary center or axis.[16] Accordingly, the lumbar vertebrae have the potential for three degrees of freedom, as motion can occur along and about three perpendicular axes (Fig. 5.1).

However, this model does not account for the anatomical factors which modify and restrict the actual motion which can occur. Clinically, the lumbosacral junction appears to exhibit two degrees of freedom of motion, flexion/extension in the sagittal plane and

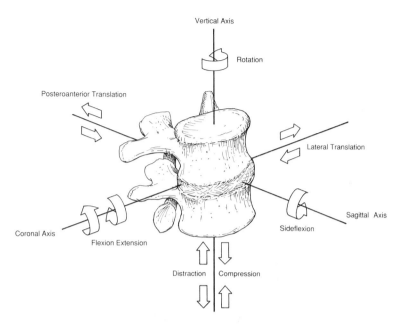

Fig. 5.1 'Potential' osteokinematic motion of the lumbar vertebrae.

rotation/sideflexion in an oblique plane. Flexion/extension is an integral part of forward/backward bending of the trunk while rotation/sideflexion occurs during any other motion of the trunk.

Flexion/extension

Segmental flexion/extension (Fig. 5.2) is the purest motion available at the lumbosacral junction and occurs during forward and backward bending of the trunk on the pelvic girdle or the pelvic girdle on the trunk. Neither rotation nor sideflexion should occur coupled with flexion/extension during forward or backward bending in the presence of a level sacral base. The coronal axis about which this motion occurs is dynamic rather than static and moves forward with flexion (Figs 5.2, 5.3).[16,44,45,137] Thus posteroanterior translation couples with flexion/extension to produce physiological forward and backward bending at the lumbosacral junction. The degree of translation at the lumbosacral junction is controlled by the iliolumbar ligaments. The results of quantitative analysis studies for flexion/extension are found in Table 5.2.

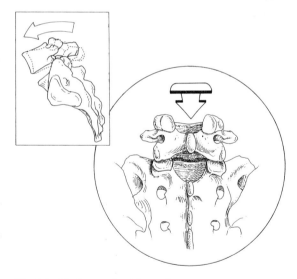

Fig. 5.2 Flexion at the L5 vertebra.

The arthrokinematics which occur during flexion and extension are impure swings. During flexion, the inferior articular processes of the L5 vertebra slide superiorly and anteriorly along the superior articular processes of the sacrum.[16] During extension, the inferior articular processes of the L5 vertebra slide

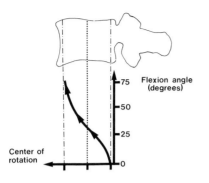

Fig. 5.3 The coronal axis for flexion/extension at the L5 vertebra moves anteriorly with increasing degrees of flexion.[44]

Table 5.2 The results of quantitative analysis studies for motion at the lumbosacral junction

	Flexion/ Extension	Rotation	Sideflexion
White[137]	20°	5°	3°
Lumsden[74]		6°	
Gregersen[47]		12° standing 3° sitting	
Farfan[32,33]	18°–20°	3°	
Pearcy[95,96]	14°	2°	3°
Bogduk[15,16]	5°–15°	3°	

inferiorly and posteriorly along the superior articular processes of the sacrum.

Rotation/sideflexion

Mechanical coupling of motion of the vertebral column during rotation and/or lateral bending of the trunk was first recorded by Lovett[72] in 1903. He noted that a flexible rod bent in one plane could not be bent in another without twisting. Unfortunately, some researchers appear to have ignored this physiological fact in attempting to analyse *pure* axial rotation about a vertical axis and *pure* sideflexion about a sagittal axis while discounting the consequential coupled motions which tended to occur.[74,95,96] This has lead to a wide variety of both qualitative (Table 5.3) and quantitative (Table 5.2) findings of segmental motion. Table 5.3 documents the qualitative findings of a few investigators with respect to the direction of mechanica

Table 5.3 The direction of mechanical coupling of rotation/sideflexion of the L5–S1 segment when either motion is introduced from a position of flexion, neutral or extension

	Flexion	Neutral	Extension
Lovett[72]	Same	Opposite	Same
MacConnaill[76]	Same	Not stated	Opposite
Kaltenborn[48]	Same	Not stated	Same
Grieve[48]	Same	Not stated	Opposite
Evejnth[30]	Same	Not stated	Opposite
Pearcy[95,96]	Same	Not stated	Same
Gracovetsky[44,45]	Opposite	Not stated	Opposite

coupling of sideflexion and rotation of the L5–S1 segment when either motion is introduced from a position of flexion, neutral or extension. A discrepancy is readily noted.

Recently, the coupled kinematic motion which occurs during axial rotation or lateral bending of the trunk has been described.[14] The motion is *unidirectional* about an oblique axis (Fig. 5.4); there is no standard name for this motion. The superior vertebra slightly flexes and sideflexes in the opposite direction to the rotation. *This is not the combination of three separate motions* but rather one movement about one axis described in known terminology. Unfortunately, this study,[44] does not specify whether or not the osteokinematic motion of the lumbosacral junction during axial rotation or lateral bending is consistent with those segments above the L5 vertebra.

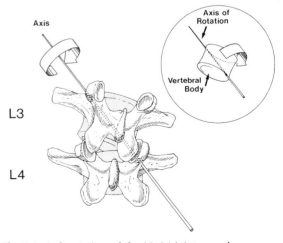

Fig. 5.4 Left rotation of the L3–L4 joint complex.

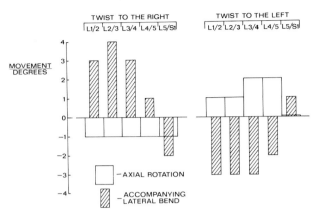

MOVEMENT DEGREES

□ — AXIAL ROTATION

▨ — ACCOMPANYING LATERAL BEND

Fig. 5.5 Findings[96] of coupled motion of rotation and lateral bending in the lumbar spine. At the lumbosacral junction, lateral bending occurs in the same direction as the induced rotation. (Redrawn from Pearcy & Tibrewal 1984.)[96]

Clinically, they do not appear to be synonymous.

In 1984, Pearcy[96] reported on a three-dimensional radiographic study of lumbar motion during rotation and lateral bending of 10 men under 30 years of age. The findings of coupled motion in this study (Fig. 5.5) were consistent with those of Gracovetsky[44] except at the lumbosacral junction where 'if lateral bending occurred, it was always in the same direction as the axial rotation'[96] (Fig. 5.6). The L4–L5 joint complex was noted to be transitional following

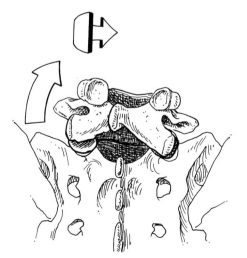

Fig. 5.6 During right rotation, the L5 vertebra rotates/sideflexes to the right.

the movement pattern of either L3–L4 or L5–S1. Perhaps the attachments of the iliolumbar ligament are influential here. Rotation/lateral bending was very restricted at the lumbosacral junction when compared to the other levels, again perhaps due to the iliolumbar ligaments.[96]

The biomechanics of the lumbosacral junction have been shown[32,40,51,65,67,112,124,137] to change with both age and degeneration. The instantaneous center of rotation for flexion/extension and/or rotation/sideflexion can be significantly displaced with degeneration, resulting in excessive posteroanterior and/or lateral translation during physiological motion of the trunk.[112,137] Consequently, 'on the intersegmental level . . . normal loads may in fact be acting about a displaced IAR [instantaneous axis of rotation], thus locally producing abnormal motion'.[40]

In summary, even if the biomechanics of the lumbosacral junction were confirmed and conclusive, the potential for altered biomechanics to exist is high, rendering 'perceptive clinical observation of a patient [as] the most direct way to assess spine motion clinically, despite its lack of objectivity'.[112] Flexion/extension of the lumbosacral junction during forward/backward bending of the trunk and/or the pelvic girdle requires the total excursion of available arthrokinematic motion and clinically yields the greatest amount of information with respect to articular mobility when assessed both actively and passively (see Ch. 7).

LUMBOSACRAL JUNCTION—KINETICS

The kinetic analysis of the lumbosacral junction pertains to the study of the anatomical factors which resist compression, torsion and posteroanterior shear of the L5 vertebra on the sacrum.

Compression

Compression of an object results when two forces act towards each other (see Fig.

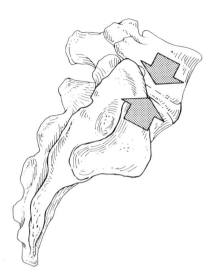

Fig. 5.7 Compression of the lumbosacral junction.

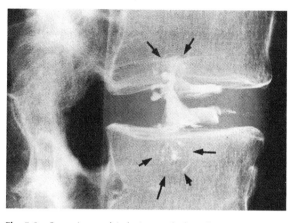

Fig. 5.8 Superior and inferior end-plate fractures (Schmorl's nodes) detected via a discogram. Note the penetration of the dye into both the superior and inferior vertebral bodies through the end-plate (arrows). (Reproduced with permission from Farfan 1973.)[32]

5.1). The main restraint to compression at the lumbosacral junction is the vertebral body/annulus-nucleus unit, although the zygapophysial joints of the L5–S1 segment have been noted[32,44,45,65] to support up to 20% of the axial compression load (Fig. 5.7). Both the annulus and the nucleus transmit the load to the end-plate of the vertebral body. The thin cortical shell of the vertebral body provides the bulk of the compression strength, being simultaneously supported by a hydraulic mechanism within the cancellous core, the contribution of which is dependent upon the rate of loading. When compression is applied slowly, fluid is squeezed out of the cancellous core via the veins; however, when the rate of compression is increased, the small vessel size may retard the rate of outflow such that the internal pressure of the vertebral body rises, thus increasing the compressive strength of the unit. In this manner, the vertebral body supports and protects the intervertebral disc against compression overload. The anatomical structure which initially yields to high loads of compression is the hyaline cartilage of the end-plate. The fracture appears radiographically as a Schmorl's node (Fig. 5.8).[32,44,45,65,67] This lesion is commonly seen at the higher lumbar levels as opposed to the lumbosacral junction.

Torsion

When a force is applied to an object at any location other than the center of rotation, it will cause the object to rotate about an axis through this pivot point. The magnitude of the torque force can be calculated by multiplying the quantity of the force applied by the distance the force acts from the pivot. Axial torsion of the L5 vertebra occurs when the bone rotates about a vertical axis through the center of the body (Fig. 5.9) and is resisted by anatomical factors located within the vertebral arch namely the:[44]

1. osseous impaction of the zygapophysial joint on the opposite side of the direction of axial rotation
2. capsular distraction of the zygapophysial joint on the same side as the direction of axial rotation
3. interspinous and supraspinous ligaments
4. anterior, posterior and superior bands of the iliolumbar ligament
5. segmental spinal musculature
as well as the structures of the vertebral body/intervertebral disc unit namely the:
6. anterior longitudinal ligament
7. outer annular fibers of the intervertebral disc
8. posterior longitudinal ligament.

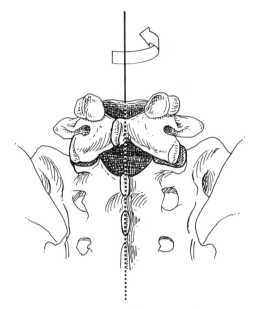

Fig. 5.9 Right axial torsion of the L5 vertebra is resisted by osseous impaction of the left zygapophysial joint and capsular distraction of the right zygapophysial joint as well as the segmental ligaments, the intervertebral disc and the myofascia.

Anatomically, the superior articular process of the sacrum (see Fig. 4.2) is squat and strong as opposed to the inferior articular process of the L5 vertebra which is much longer and receives less support from the pedicle. Consequently, the inferior process is more easily deflected when the zygapophysial joint is loaded at 90° to its articular surface. This process can deflect 8° to 9° medially during axial torsion beyond which trabecular fractures and residual strain deformation will occur.[32,44]

The structure and orientation of the annular fibers is critical to the ability of the intervertebral disc to resist torsion. 'The concentric arrangement of the collagenous layers of the annulus ensures that when the disk is placed in tension, shear or rotation, the individual fibers are always in tension'.[65] Under static loading conditions, injuries occur with as little as 2° and certainly by 3.5° of axial rotation.[44] The iliolumbar ligament (see Figs 4.12, 4.15) plays an important role in minimizing torque forces at the lumbosacral junction. The longer

the transverse process of the L5 vertebra and consequently the shorter the iliolumbar ligament, the stronger the segment is to torsion.[32]

Axial compression also increases the segmental torque strength by 35%.[44] During forward flexion of the lumbar spine, the instantaneous center of rotation moves forward (see Fig. 5.3) thus increasing the compressive load and consequently the ability of the joint to resist torsion.[32,44] Clinically, this becomes very important when re-educating lumbo-pelvic-hip ergonomics (see Ch. 11).

The degree of lumbar curve, or lordosis, is of extreme importance for the individual. The curve itself is structured by the wedging of the discs, particularly at L4, by the wedging of the vertebral bodies, and by the obliquity of the upper surface of the body of the sacrum. When this curve is reduced, as in forward flexion, the range of lateral flexion is much reduced or even zeroed. Thus, asymmetric erector spinae activity will not produce appreciable axial rotation. Because the axis of rotation is moved forward in the flexed position, the resistance to torsion offered by the facets is increased. The amount of axial torsion induced by lateral bending increases as the lumbar curve is reconstituted as it extends from the flexed position. It is therefore of extreme importance to control the lordosis in flexion–extension.[44]

Posteroanterior shear

Shear occurs when an applied force produces sliding between two planes (see Fig. 5.1). Posteroanterior shear at the lumbosacral junction occurs when a force attempts to displace the L5 vertebra anterior to the sacrum (Fig. 5.10). The anatomical factors which resist posteroanterior shear at the lumbosacral junction are primarily the impaction of the inferior articular processes of the L5 vertebra against the superior articular processes of the sacrum and the iliolumbar ligaments. Secondary factors include the intervertebral disc, the anterior longitudinal ligament, the posterior longitudinal ligament and the midline posterior ligamentous system.[32,65,123]

Dynamically, the posterior midline ligaments and the thoracolumbar fascia are important in balancing the anterior shear

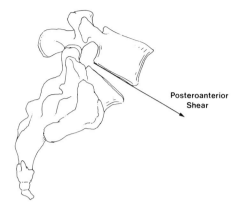

Fig. 5.10 Posteroanterior shear of the L5 vertebra on the sacrum.

forces which occur when large loads are lifted.[16,44] The optimal method of loading the spine should balance both compression and shear such that the magnitude of the resultant force does not exceed the strength of the joint. Consequently, both the articular and the myofascial components are required to balance the moment of a large external load. 'We have found that for any load, for minimum equalized stress, there is a privileged stable zone corresponding to the situation in which the moment will be balanced and shared in equal thirds by muscle, midline ligament system, and by the abdominals through the thoracolumbar fascia'.[44]

PELVIC GIRDLE—KINEMATICS

Even though mobility of the sacroiliac joint has been recognized since the 17th century, specific biomechanical analysis of this articulation has received very little disciplined attention. In 1878, Meyer[87] described two kinds of sacral 'rocking' both occurring about a transverse axis, one within the articular surface and the other 1 cm posterior to the second sacral vertebral body. Both motions were thought to accompany forward and backward bending of the trunk. Various axes of sacral and/or innominate bone motion have since been proposed[88,89] (Fig. 5.11) some with, and others without, scientific validation.

The methods used in kinematic research of the pelvic girdle include:
1. manual manipulation of the sacroiliac joint both at surgery and in a cadaver[21,35,59]
2. X-ray analysis in various postures of the trunk and lower extremity[4,20]
3. sterioradiographs[28]
4. inclinometer measurements in various postures of the trunk and lower extremity after the insertion of Kirschner wires into the innominate bone and sacrum.[98]

The results of these studies has led to proposals of both osteokinematic and arthrokinematic function of the pelvic girdle.

The following section will detail the current status on both the known and the proposed

Axes

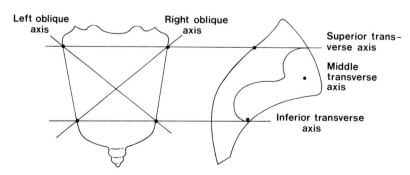

Fig. 5.11 The various axes about which motion of the sacrum and/or innominate bones have been proposed.[88,89] (Redrawn from Mitchell 1965.)[88]

biomechanics of the pelvic girdle from which a logical examination and treatment protocol can be developed.

Osteokinematics

Osteokinematics refers to the study of motion of bones regardless of the motion of the joints. In this respect, the pelvic girdle as a unit is capable of motion in all three body planes. It has the ability to:
1. bend forward and backward in the sagittal plane—flex/extend
2. bend laterally to the left and right in the coronal plane
3. rotate axially to the left and right in the transverse plane.

Forward and backward bending in the sagittal plane

Forward bending.   Forward bending from the erect standing position (Fig. 5.12) results in a posterior displacement of the proximal femora, thus shifting the center of gravity behind the pedal base. Simultaneously, the pelvic girdle as a unit flexes on the femoral heads while the thoracolumbar column forward bends in a superoinferior direction until the L5 vertebra flexes forward on the sacrum.

Following this, the sacrum flexes between the two innominate bones with no apparent rotation or lateral bending. Simultaneously, the two innominate bones rotate about an antero-posterior oblique axis such that the iliac crests and the PSISs approximate while the ischial tuberosities and the ASISs separate (Fig. 5.13).[22,27,88,134,135] Clinically, the opposite rotation of the innominate bone has also been observed.[130] The direction of rotation is possibly dependent upon the anteroposterior dimension of the sacrum (S1 to S3) in the transverse plane (see Ch. 4).

Once the sacrum becomes locked between the two innominate bones, the pelvic girdle as a unit continues to flex forward on the posteriorly translating femoral heads. This motion results in the smooth transference of the body weight posterior to the pedal base, thus maintaining stability and balance. The order in which these motions occur can be varied at will; however, when the axial skeleton is significantly compressed, the above described biomechanics are optimal.

Backward bending. Backward bending from the erect standing position (Fig. 5.14) results in an anterior displacement of the proximal femora, thus shifting the center of gravity in front of the pedal base. Simultaneously, the pelvic girdle as a unit extends on the femoral

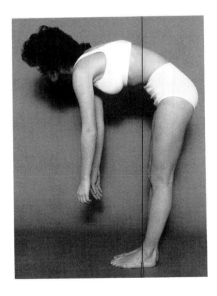 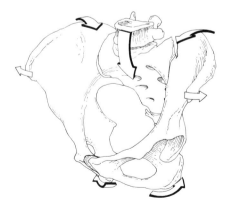

Figs 5.12 and 5.13 Forward bending of the trunk from the erect standing position, and the osteokinematic motion of the pelvic girdle.

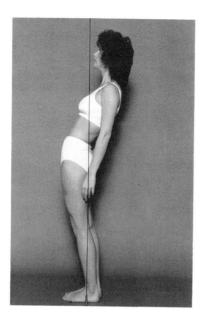
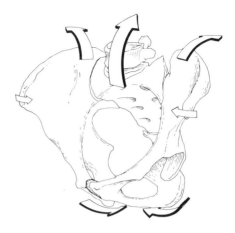

Figs 5.14 and 5.15 Backward bending of the trunk from the erect standing position, and the osteokinematic motion of the pelvic girdle.

heads while the thoracolumbar spine extends in a superoinferior direction until the L5 vertebra extends backward on the sacrum.

Following this, the sacrum extends between the two innominate bones which simultaneously rotate about an anteroposterior oblique axis such that the iliac crests and the PSISs separate while the ischial tuberosities and the ASISs approximate (Fig. 5.15). Clinically, the opposite rotation of the innominate bone has also been observed, possibly reflecting the variable anteroposterior dimension of the sacrum in the transverse plane.[130]

Once the sacrum becomes locked between the two innominate bones, the pelvic girdle as a unit continues to extend backward on the anteriorly translating femoral heads, thus resulting in further bilateral femoral extension. As with forward bending, the order in which these motions occur can be varied at will; however, the above described biomechanics are optimal.

Lateral bending in the coronal plane

Lateral bending of the pelvic girdle in the coronal plane is an unphysiological motion when static. In locomotion, it becomes an integral part of rapid lateral motion and is an extremely useful movement to assess in the clinic. Hence the need for detailed knowledge of the underlying osteokinematics.

Left lateral bending. Left lateral bending from the erect standing position (Fig. 5.16) is initiated by displacement of the femora to the right, thus maintaining the line of gravity central within the pedal base.[70] Subsequently, the pelvic girdle *as a unit* sidebends to the left on the translating femoral heads, resulting in adduction of the right femur and abduction of the left femur. *Within the pelvic girdle itself*, intra-pelvic torsion occurs. During this motion, the right innominate bone posteriorly rotates relative to the anteriorly rotating left innominate bone, while the sacrum rotates to the right about an oblique axis (Fig. 5.17).

Pitkin and Pheasant,[98] using inclinometer measurements and lateral radiographs, noted that the innominate bones were the moving members during lateral bending and rotation and that the sacrum followed passively. With respect to the sacrum, 'It should be emphasized that lateral bending and rotation normally do not occur alone, but as correlated movements, and that in this respect the sacrum does not differ from the rest of the presacral vertebrae'.[98] Right rotation of the sacrum between the two innominate bones

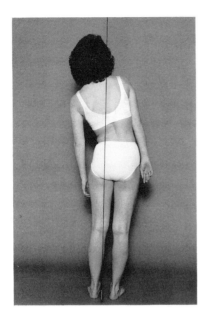

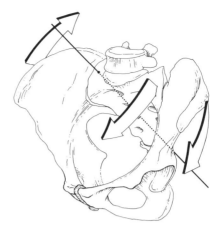

Figs 5.16 and 5.17 Left lateral bending of the trunk. The osteokinematic motion of the pelvic girdle comprises posterior rotation of the right innominate bone, anterior rotation of the left innominate bone and right rotation of the sacrum.

results in a deepening of the left sacral sulcus, an anterior displacement of the left sacral base, a shallowing of the right sacral sulcus, a posterior displacement of the right sacral base, a posterior displacement of the right inferior lateral angle of the sacrum, and an anterior displacement of the left inferior lateral angle of the sacrum (Fig. 5.18). These osteokinematic motions reflect the obliquity of sacral rotation during antagonistic motion of the innominate bones (Fig. 5.17).

The L5 vertebra rotates/sideflexes to the right, *relative to the sacrum*, about a postero-anterior oblique axis. Note that the rotation of the L5 vertebra follows that of the sacrum as well as the posteriorly rotating innominate bone.

Axial rotation in the transverse plane

Axial rotation of the pelvic girdle, together with axial rotation of the vertebral column, knees and feet, allows the eyes to scan 360° from a stationary point. During left axial rotation, the femora twist to the left about a midline vertical axis, resulting in an antero-medial displacement of the proximal right femur and a posteromedial displacement of the proximal left femur. Simultaneously, the

pelvic girdle as a unit rotates to the left on the displaced femoral heads, resulting in extension and lateral rotation of the right femur and flexion and medial rotation of the left femur. The twist continues in an inferosuperior direction, producing intra-pelvic torsion. The right innominate bone anteriorly rotates while the left innominate bone posteriorly rotates. Both

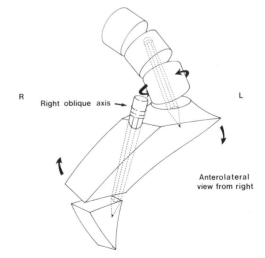

R

Right oblique axis →

L

Anterolateral view from right

Fig. 5.18 Right rotation of the sacrum and right rotation/sideflexion of the L5 vertebra secondary to left lateral bending of the trunk. (Redrawn from Mitchell 1965.)[88]

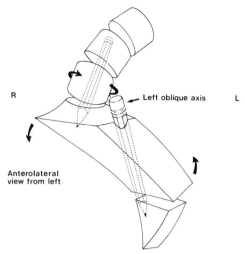

R

← Left oblique axis   L

Anterolateral
view from left

Fig. 5.19 Left rotation of the sacrum, left rotation/sideflexion of the L5 vertebra secondary to left axial rotation of the trunk. (Redrawn from Mitchell 1965.)[88]

bones passively drive the sacrum into left rotation.

Left sacral rotation between the two innominate bones results in a deepening of the right sacral sulcus, an anterior displacement of the right sacral base, a shallowing of the left sacral sulcus, a posterior displacement of the left sacral base, a posterior displacement of the left inferior lateral angle of the sacrum, and an anterior displacement of the right inferior lateral angle of the sacrum (Fig. 5.19). These osteokinematic motions again reflect the obliquity of sacral rotation which occurs subsequent to antagonistic motion of the innominate bones (Fig. 5.17).

The L5 vertebra rotates/sideflexes to the left, *relative to the sacrum*, about a postero-anterior oblique axis. Note that the rotation of the L5 vertebra follows that of the sacrum as well as the posteriorly rotating innominate bone.

Arthrokinematics

Arthrokinematics refers to the study of motion of joints regardless of the motion of the bones. The arthrokinematics of the sacroiliac joint which fulfill the osteokinematic function of the innominate bones and the sacrum are

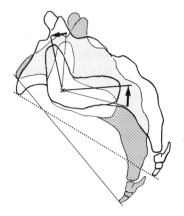

Fig. 5.20 Proposed intra-articular transverse axis of sacral rotation. (Redrawn from Kapandji 1974.)[61]

controversial. Earlier investigators[87,98] felt that sacral flexion/extension occurred about a stationary transverse axis that some felt lay within and others outside of the articular surface of the joint (Figs 5.20, 5.21). In 1954, Weisl[134] refuted these theories of sacral rotation about a fixed horizontal axis for the following reasons:

1. the arcuate groove and gutter along which the articular surfaces were proposed to slide only appear later in life
2. these sacral motions presupposed a degree of congruence between the articular surfaces which does not exist
3. overriding of the reciprocal elevations and depressions leading to a wide separation of the articular surfaces would be forced to occur.

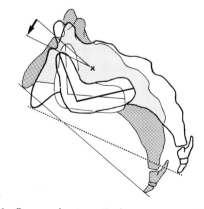

Fig. 5.21 Proposed extra-articular transverse axis of sacral rotation. (Redrawn from Kapandji 1974.)[61]

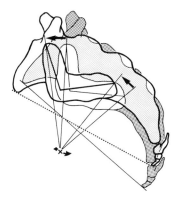

Fig. 5.22 Proposed dynamic extra-articular transverse axis of sacral rotation. (Redrawn from Kapandji 1974.)[61]

Subsequent to his motion studies, Weisl[135] concluded that the axis of motion for sacral flexion/extension lay outside of the joint approximately 10 cm inferior to the sacral promontory (Fig. 5.22) and was a moving axis of rotation. This theory would require an impure swing[76] to occur between the articular surfaces. This theory was supported by Pratt[99] who, in 1952, stated that sacral flexion required an inferior glide of the sacrum along the short arm of the articular surface together with a posterior glide along the long arm. Weisl[134] agreed that separately each sacroiliac joint could move both superoinferiorly and posteroanteriorly, but felt that when the two joints were conjoined at the pubic symphysis, only the posteroanterior movement could occur. Both Colachis,[22] in 1963, and Wilder,[138] in 1980, concluded from their studies that both angular and parallel movements of the sacrum took place rather than pure rotary motion but neither investigator detailed the specific arthrokinematics which occurred during the motions studied.

Sacral rotation has not received the same investigative study as flexion/extension and a variety of combined articular glides has been proposed[88,89] but not scientifically validated. Beal,[9] and subsequently Meadows,[81] propose that the 'sense' of sacroiliac joint motion may be due to deformation of the thick intra-articular fibrocartilage rather than specific 'sliding' of the articular surfaces.

In summary, osteokinematically the sacrum flexes, extends, and rotates to the left and right during habitual movement (forward/backward bending, lateral bending, axial rotation). The specific arthrokinematics and the axes about which these motions occur are at best hypothetical.

Antagonistic motions of the innominate bones in a parasagittal plane occur during lateral bending and axial rotation. These motions are usually referred to as anterior and posterior rotation; however, perhaps the correct terminology should be flexion/extension since elsewhere when a bone rotates about a paracoronal axis the terms flexion/extension are employed.[97]

Once again, we are left with what is known being short of ideal for dogmatic biomechanical statements of pelvic girdle dysfunction; however, with the advent of less invasive investigative techniques perhaps the next decade will yield scientific evidence of sacroiliac arthrokinematic function in the living.

PELVIC GIRDLE—KINETICS

The pelvic girdle is required to transmit the weight of the head, trunk and upper extremities to the lower extremities as well as to resist the forces incurred during motion of the lower extremities. The mechanism by which these tasks are accomplished constitutes the kinetic function of the pelvic girdle.

The pelvic girdle can be divided into two arches (Fig. 5.23), the posterior and the anterior, by the coronal plane which passes through the acetabular fossae. The function of each arch is dependent upon the structural integrity of the other.[61] The components of the posterior arch include:
1. the upper three sacral vertebrae and their contiguous joints
2. the two ilii
3. the two sacroiliac joints.
The components of the anterior arch include:
1. the two pubic bones
2. the fibrocartilaginous disc between the two pubic bones
3. the pubic symphysis.

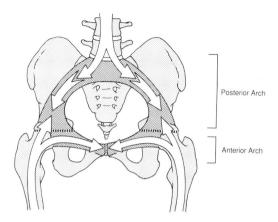

Fig. 5.23 The posterior and anterior arches of the pelvic girdle. The function of each arch is dependent upon the structural integrity of the other.

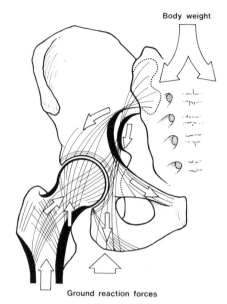

Ground reaction forces

Fig. 5.24 The orientation of the bony trabeculae within the pelvic girdle corresponds to the lines of force met in both static and dynamic function. (Redrawn from Kapandji 1970.)[60]

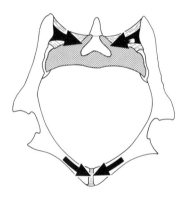

Fig. 5.25 A transverse section through the pelvic girdle illustrating the significant role the anterior arch plays in the stability of the sacroiliac joint. Anterior instability causes the innominate bones to separate thus permitting the anteroinferior displacement of the sacral promontory into the pelvic bowl.

The body weight is transferred from the L5 vertebra to the hip joint via the ala of the sacrum through the sacroiliac joint at the junction of the short and long arms and along the arcuate line to the acetabulum. Ground reaction forces which travel up the lower extremity are transmitted superiorly via the same bony trabeculae, as well as across the pubic rami, to counterbalance the ascending forces from the contralateral limb. A complex system of bony trabeculae exists within the sacrum and the innominate bones and corresponds to these lines of force (Fig. 5.24).[60] Efficient weight transference is dependent upon both the osseous and the articular stability of the posterior and anterior arches.

During erect standing there is a tendency for the superincumbent body weight to force the sacral promontory into the pelvic bowl (see Fig. 4.14). The anatomical factors which resist this torque are both osseous and articular. The anteroinferior force on the upper sacrum is resisted by the wedge shape of the upper sacral segments (see Fig. 4.5) which narrow in a superoinferior direction at S1 and S2 and in an inferosuperior direction at S3.[110] As the sacrum is forced anteroinferiorly, the innominate bones are stressed transversely at the pubic symphysis. The components of the anterior arch act as a tiebeam to prevent separation of this articulation (Fig. 5.25). If the pubic symphysis is

unstable, there is a tendency for the two innominate bones to separate thus allowing the displacement of the sacral promontory into the pelvic bowl.

Forward rotation (flexion) of the sacrum between the two innominate bones is an integral component of forward bending of the trunk and is resisted strongly by the sacrotuberous, sacrospinous, dorsal sacroiliac, interosseous ligaments and weakly by the ventral sacroiliac ligament (see Fig. 4.14). In health, the osseous and ligamentous restraining mechanism functions optimally to prevent excessive motion of either the innominate or the sacral bones. Colachis[22] has noted that 400 to 2600 pound-force (1780–11570 N) are necessary to disrupt the pelvic girdle and feels that an inherent weakness must exist for instability to occur.

The angle of inclination (see Figs 4.6, 4.7, 4.8) of the articular surface of the sacrum is a significant factor in the inherent stability of the sacroiliac joint.[110] Vertically oriented sacroiliac joints (Type B) subject the ligaments to greater stress since less of the load is borne by the osseous components of the posterior arch. Asymmetric loading of the sacroiliac joint may occur in the presence of structural asymmetry of the angle of inclination (Type C—Fig. 5.26; see also Fig. 4.8), or postural asymmetry (short leg). Again, this increased load is borne by the sacroiliac ligaments.

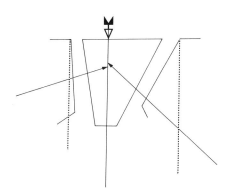

Fig. 5.26 Asymmetric loading of the sacroiliac joints occurs if the angle of inclination of the articular surface is asymmetric.

The angle of inclination also determines the proportion of the articular surface which bears the load and is influenced by the posture of the sacrum. The more vertical the sacrum, the more the articular surface participates in weight transference, thus reducing the stress on the ligamentous system. Kinetically, this supports the practice of teaching lifting in a posture of pelvic tilt (see Ch. 5—lifting; Ch. 11).

Pregnancy

The pelvic girdle has been shown [19,52,131,142] to exhibit excessive mobility secondary to relaxation of the ligaments of the sacroiliac joints and the pubic symphysis during pregnancy. This process begins during the 4th month and continues until the 7th month of pregnancy, following which only a slight increase in mobility occurs. Great variation in the degree of both transverse and superoinferior widening of the pubic symphysis has been noted radiologically,[19,52] with the average increase being 5 mm.

According to Hagen, relaxation of the pelvic girdle in pregnancy is due to the presence of a specific high molecular-weight hormone, relaxin, which together with oestrogen causes 'depolymerization of hyaluronic acid . . . Compressive, shearing and tensile forces constitute a chronic trauma increasing the concentration of hyaluronidase . . . This interferes with the humoral conditions needed for pelvic stability and very likely also plays a certain role as a pathogenetic factor in pelvic relaxation'.[52]

Consequently, the locking mechanism of the pelvic girdle is less effective, thus increasing the strain on the ligaments of both the sacroiliac joints and the pubic symphysis. The morphological changes within the pelvic girdle associated with pregnancy are universal and often occur without symptoms. Occasionally, women present between the 26th and 28th weeks with increasing tenderness over the sacroiliac joint and/or pubic symphysis secondary to loss of kinetic function. Normally, the pelvic girdle returns to its prepregnant state between the 3rd and 6th month postpartum and simply requires external stabilization during this period (see Ch. 9). Rarely, one innominate bone may rotate and lock on the sacrum virtually 'subluxing' the sacroiliac joint, requiring a manipulative reduction for recovery.

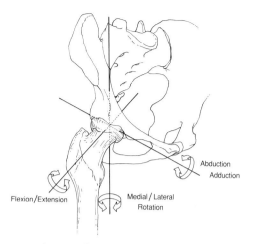

Flexion/Extension

Abduction
Adduction

Medial / Lateral
Rotation

Fig. 5.27 The osteokinematic motion of the femur.

HIP—KINEMATICS

The femur articulates with the innominate bone via a ball-and-socket joint, the hip, which is capable of circumductive motion. The hip is classified as an unmodified ovoid joint and is capable of three degrees of freedom of motion about three perpendicular axes (Fig. 5.27).[76] Rotation of the femur about these three axes produces the motions commonly known as:
1. flexion/extension
2. abduction/adduction
3. medial/lateral rotation.

Flexion/extension (osteokinematics) occurs when either the pelvic girdle as a unit or the free femur rotates about a coronal axis through the center of the femoral head and neck. Approximately 100° of femoral flexion is possible, following which motion of the sacro-iliac and intervertebral joints occurs to allow the anterior thigh to approximate the chest.[131] Approximately 20° of femoral extension is possible.[60] When rotation of the femoral head occurs purely about this axis (i.e. without conjoined abduction/adduction or medial/lateral rotation) the motion is described as a pure spin (arthrokinematics).

Abduction/adduction (osteokinematics) occurs when either the pelvic girdle as a unit or the free femur rotates about a sagittal axis through the center of the femoral head.

Approximately 45° of femoral abduction and 30° of femoral adduction are possible, following which the pelvic girdle laterally bends beneath the vertebral column.[60] When the femur rotates purely about this sagittal axis the head of the femur transcribes a supero-inferior chord within the acetabulum (i.e. the shortest distance between two points), therefore this motion is described as a pure swing (arthrokinematics).

Medial/lateral rotation (osteokinematics) occurs when either the pelvic girdle as a unit or the free femur rotates about a longitudinal axis. The location of this axis is dependent upon fixation of the foot. When the pelvic girdle rotates about a firmly planted foot, the longitudinal axis of rotation runs from the center of the femoral head through to the lateral femoral condyle. When the foot is off the ground, the femur can rotate about a variety of longitudinal axes all of which pass through the femoral head and the foot.[131] Approximately 30° to 40° of medial rotation and 60° of lateral rotation are possible.[60] Pure femoral rotation about this axis causes the femoral head to transcribe an anteroposterior chord within the acetabulum and arthrokine-matically this motion is described as a pure swing.

Habitual movement of the femur relative to the innominate bone does not produce pure arthrokinematic motion. Rather, a combination of movement patterns are the norm. Osteokinematically, the habitual pattern of motion for the non-weight-bearing lower extremity is a combination of (a) flexion, abduction and lateral rotation, with (b) extension, adduction and medial rotation. Arthro-kinematically, both motions are impure swings. During gait, the movement pattern consists of femoral flexion, adduction and lateral rotation, followed by extension, abduction and medial rotation which arthrokine-matically are impure swings as well.

HIP—KINETICS

The hip is subjected to forces equal to mul-tiples of the body weight and requires osseous, articular and myofascial integrity for stability. The factors which contribute to stability at the hip include:

1. the anatomical configuration of the joint as well as the orientation of the trabeculae
2. the strength and orientation of the capsule and the ligaments during habitual movements
3. the strength of the periarticular muscles and fascia.

During erect standing, the superincumbent body weight is distributed equally through the pelvic girdle to the femoral heads and necks. Each hip joint supports approximately 33% of the body weight which subsequently produces a bending moment between the neck of the femur and its shaft.[109] A complex system of bony trabeculae exists within the femoral head and neck to prevent superoinferior shearing of the femoral head during erect standing (Fig. 5.24).[60]

The orientation of the capsule and the articular ligaments (see Figs 4.19, 4.20) also contributes to stability at the hip during habitual motion (Table 5.4). Extension of the femur winds all of the extra-articular ligaments around the femoral neck and renders them taut. The inferior band of the iliofemoral ligament is under the greatest tension in exten-

sion. Flexion of the femur unwinds the extra-articular ligaments, and when combined with slight adduction, predisposes the femoral head to posterior dislocation if sufficient force is applied to the distal end of the femur (e.g. dashboard impact).

During lateral rotation of the femur, the iliotrochanteric band of the iliofemoral ligament and the pubofemoral ligament become taut while the ischiofemoral ligament becomes slack. Conversely, during medial rotation of the femur, the anterior ligaments become slack while the ischiofemoral ligament becomes taut.

Abduction of the femur tenses the pubofemoral ligament, the inferior band of the iliofemoral ligament as well as the ischiofemoral ligament. At the end of abduction, the neck of the femur impacts onto the acetabular rim thus distorting and everting the labrum.[60] In this manner, the acetabular labrum deepens the articular cavity thus increasing stability without limiting mobility. Adduction results in tension of the iliotrochanteric band of the iliofemoral ligament while the others remain relatively slack.

The ligamentum teres is under moderate tension in erect standing as well as during medial and lateral rotation of the femur. Kapandji[60] notes that the acetabular fossa outlines the extreme positions of the foveal attachment of the ligamentum teres during habitual motion.

The bones and ligaments are not alone in the maintenance of stability at the hip. They receive dynamic support from the multiple muscles which cross and also attach to the capsule of the hip joint. Standing on one limb dramatically increases the magnitude of forces which must be met at the hip joint (2.4 to 2.6 times the body weight) and subsequently requires recruitment of the periarticular muscles for maintenance of equilibrium. The body weight must be shifted such that the line of gravity falls through the supporting limb distally. The force developed by the muscle contraction multiplied by length of the lateral lever arm to the joint axis must be balanced by the force developed by the body weight

Table 5.4 Resultant tension of the extra-articular ligaments of the hip joint during motion of the femur

Femoral motion	Ligament	Tension
Extension	All extra-articular ligaments	Taut
Flexion/adduction	All ligaments	Slack
Lateral rotation	Iliotrochanteric	Taut
	Pubofemoral	Taut
	Ischiofemoral	Slack
Medial rotation	Iliofemoral	Slack
	Pubofemoral	Slack
	Ischiofemoral	Taut
Abduction	Pubofemoral	Taut
	Inferior band*	Taut
	Ischiofemoral	Taut
	Iliotrochanteric	Slack
Adduction	Iliotrochanteric	Taut
	Inferior band*	Slack
	Ischiofemoral	Slack
	Pubofemoral	Slack

* Inferior band of iliofemoral ligament

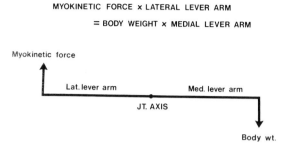

MYOKINETIC FORCE x LATERAL LEVER ARM

= BODY WEIGHT x MEDIAL LEVER ARM

Fig. 5.28 The kinetic forces medial and lateral to the axis of the hip joint must be equal if balance is to be preserved.

multiplied by the length of the medial lever arm to the joint axis if balance is to be preserved (Fig. 5.28). Consequently, one legged stance can be a useful clinical test of kinetic function of the hip joint.

MYOKINEMATICS AND MYOKINETICS

Myokinematics pertains to the study of motion of bones subsequent to a muscular contraction and follows the laws of approximation and detorsion.[76,131] The resultant osteokinematic motion is dependent upon both the internal and external resistances (including gravity) met by the muscular contraction. Myokinetics pertains to the study of transarticular forces (compression, torsion, shear) produced as a consequence of muscular contraction.

Each muscle attaching to the lumbo-pelvic-hip complex elicits a specific myokinematic response which has been determined via geometric analysis and electromyographic studies.[7,131] However, habitual motion requires integrated synergistic function of a number of muscles at any one time for any one movement. These movement patterns are set neurologically and result in efficient static posture and locomotion when function is optimal. This section lists the myokinematic function of the muscles attaching to the lumbo-pelvic-hip complex (Table 5.5) and describes the integrated muscle activity which occurs during static erect standing as well as lifting.

Erect standing

It has been shown[7] that among the mammals man has the most efficient posture in bipedal stance. In the lumbo-pelvic-hip region intermittent bursts of activity from the gluteus medius, tensor fascia lata and hamstring muscles are required to control postural sway. Constant activity has been reported[7] in the iliopsoas muscle to support the iliofemoral ligament of the hip joint, as well as in the internal oblique muscle to protect the inguinal canal. All other muscle groups are quiescent when bipedal posture is optimal. Deviation from this economical position results in the immediate recruitment of both the trunk and femoral musculature, thus dramatically increasing the energy expenditure of standing still.

The transference of body weight from bipedal to unipedal stance requires coordinated facilitation and inhibition of specific muscle groups which are functions of the articular reflexes (i.e. input from the Type I and II mechanoreceptors).[140] One-legged stance requires stabilization of the pelvic girdle in the coronal plane and consequently recruits the ipsilateral gluteus medius/minimus and tensor fascia lata muscles immediately. The ipsilateral hip abductors are facilitated reflexly by the Type III mechanoreceptors located in the ligamentum teres; these reflexes are discharged following compression of the femoral head into the acetabular fossa.[26]

Lifting

Incorrect lifting technique is often responsible for initiating breakdown within the lumbo-pelvic-hip region. Consequently, education with respect to 'safe' lifting methods is paramount to the rehabilitative process (see Ch. 11). However, two diametric schools of thought have been proposed with respect to the safest method of performing a lift.[5,34,44,121] One school advocates[34,44] lifting in lumbar flexion (pelvic tilt) while the other promotes[5,121] lifting in lumbar extension. The lumbo-pelvic-

Table 5.5 The specific myokinematic function of the major muscles with respect to lumbo-pelvic-hip biomechanics

Muscle	Site	Function
Abdominals	Trunk	Flexor, rotator
Erector Spinae	Sacrum	Flexor[89]
Lumbar Iliocostalis		
Lumbar Longissimus		
unilateral	(L4) L5	Segmental rotator[11,15,16]
bilateral	(L4) L5	Extensor and retractor (prevents anterior shear)
Multifidus	Sacrum	Flexor[89]
		Segmental stabilizer 2° to increased compression[11]
Iliacus	Sacrum	Flexor[89]
	Femur	Flexor[7,54,60,131]
Gluteus Maximus	Sacrum	Extensor[89]
	Femur	Extensor[7,31,54,60,131]
cranial fibers	Femur	Abductor[7,31,60,131]
posterior fibers	Femur	Lateral rotator[7,31,54,60]
Piriformis		
bilateral	Sacrum	Extensor[89]
unilateral	Femur	Abductor[31,60,131]
		Lateral rotator[31,54,60,131]
Coccygeus	Sacrum	Extensor[89]
Quadratus Lumborum		
unilateral	Lumbar	Lateral flexor[61]
Psoas		
unilateral	Lumbar	Ipsilateral lateral flexor
		Contralateral rotator[61]
	Femur	Flexor[7,31,54,60,131]
bilateral	Pelvic girdle	Flexor on femora while extensor lumbar spine[7,60,131]
	Lumbo-pelvic-hip complex	Constant activity[7] during erect standing
Sartorius	Femur	Flexor[7,54,60,131]
		Abductor[54,131]
		Lateral rotator[54,131]
Rectus Femoris	Femur	Flexor[7,54,60,131]
Gluteus Medius/Minimus	Femur	Abductor[7,54,60,131]
anterior fibers	Femur	Flexor[60]
	Femur	Medial rotator[7,54,60,131]
posterior fibers	Femur	Extensor[60]
	Femur	Lateral rotator[60]
Hamstrings	Femur	Servile extensors[7,54,60]
Semimembranosus	Femur	Adductor[60]
Semitendinosus		Medial rotator[131]
Biceps femoris	Femur	Lateral rotator[7,131]
Tensor Fascia Lata	Femur	Medial rotator[7,54,60,131]
anterior fibers	Femur	Abductor[7,54,60,131]
Adductor Magnus	Femur	Adductor[7,54,60,131]
posterior fibers	Femur	Lateral rotator[60]
Gracilis	Femur	Adductor[54,60,131]
Quadratus Femoris	Femur	Adductor[60]
	Femur	Lateral rotator[54,60,131]
Pectineus	Femur	Adductor[54,60,131]
	Femur	Lateral rotator[60]
	Femur	Flexor[54,131]
Obturator Internus	Femur	Adductor[60]
	Femur	Lateral rotator[54,60,131]
Obturator Externus	Femur	Adductor[60]
	Femur	Lateral rotator[54,60,131]
Adductor Longus	Femur	Servile adductor[7,54,60]
	Femur	Flexor[54,131]
Adductor Brevis	Femur	Adductor[54,60]
Gemelli	Femur	Lateral rotator[54,131]
	Femur	Abductor[131]

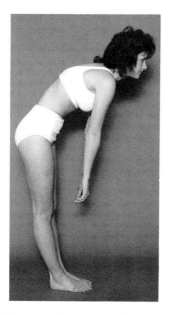

Fig. 5.29 (**left**) At 45° of anterior inclination of the trunk, the posterior ligamentous system becomes taut and the eccentric activity of the spinal extensor muscles ceases.

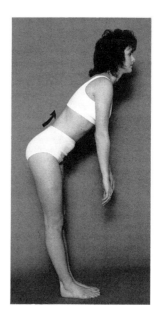

Fig. 5.30 (**right**) This movement pattern for forward bending (i.e. anterior rotation of the pelvic girdle prior to spinal flexion) is commonly seen amongst dancers and in aerobics classes.

hip arthrokinetics as well as the myokinetics strongly favor the 'pelvic tilt' position as the optimal posture for compression loading. The reasons for this will be outlined below.

Moving an object from the floor to a higher surface initially requires forward bending of the trunk. Spinal flexion is controlled by the eccentric contraction of the thoracolumbar spinal extensors. Once the trunk is inclined 45° forward, the posterior ligamentous system becomes taut and the contraction of the spinal extensors ceases (Fig. 5.29).[32] Further forward bending induces sacral flexion between the innominate bones (Fig. 5.13) (limited by the sacrotuberous and the dorsal sacroiliac ligaments and controlled eccentrically by the biceps femoris muscles) and subsequent flexion of the entire pelvic girdle on the femoral heads (controlled eccentrically by the hamstring muscles).

When the spine is not under additional compression (i.e. no weight in the arms) the sequence of forward bending can be varied at will such that anterior rotation of the pelvic girdle may occur prior to spinal flexion (Fig.

5.30). In this instance, continued isometric contraction of the thoracolumbar spinal extensors is required well beyond 45° of anterior inclination of the trunk since the posterior ligamentous system remains slack and therefore ineffectual in supporting a load. This movement pattern is commonly seen amongst dancers and in aerobics classes and if repeated often enough can become the individual's habitual movement pattern for forward bending.

As the external load increases, this altered movement pattern becomes less desirable since muscles are required to perform functions for which they are not ideally suited.[33] 'When the weightlifting strategy is changed from ligament to muscle, compression is increased for large angles of flexion. The ideal must be the use of ligament whenever possible, and this can best be done by maintaining the spine in flexion'.[44]

Kinetically, the moment of the external load is reduced if the distance between the lifted object and the vertebral column is shortened. Thus a flexible spine has the mechanical

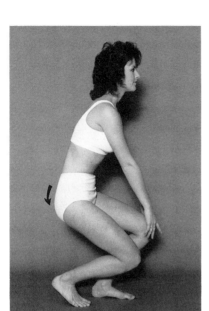

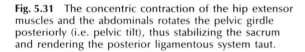

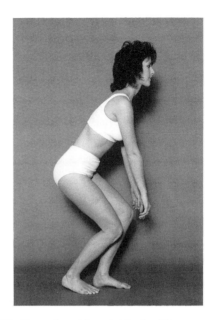

Fig. 5.31 The concentric contraction of the hip extensor muscles and the abdominals rotates the pelvic girdle posteriorly (i.e. pelvic tilt), thus stabilizing the sacrum and rendering the posterior ligamentous system taut.

Fig. 5.32 The vulnerable point in the lift occurs when the thoracolumbar spine begins to extend via the concentric activity of the spinal extensors.

advantage of reducing the distance between the shoulders and the hips thus decreasing the external load.

Returning to erect standing is initiated by backward pelvic rotation (pelvic tilt) produced by the concentric contraction of the hip extensor muscles as well as the abdominals (Fig. 5.31). This action stabilizes the sacrum between the innominate bones by tightening the sacrotuberous ligaments. As well, spinal flexion is induced, thus rendering the posterior ligamentous system taut. The weight is then lifted by further concentric contraction of the hip joint extensors. 'These muscles act on the pelvis and sacrum and are the principal muscles used to maintain the position of the pelvic girdle in relation to moments induced by external loads, lumbar muscle activities, and ligament tension on the spine'.[44]

The gluteus maximus muscle has a considerable mechanical advantage in man as compared to other primates given the increased antero-posterior depth of man's pelvis.[34] As well, more than one half of the muscle inserts into the iliotibial band distally which increases its

leverage on the hip joint, especially when the band is taut. The size and anatomy of this muscle render it an excellent 'lifter'.

As the trunk resumes its erect posture, the thoracolumbar spine begins to extend via concentric activity of the spinal extensors (Fig. 5.32). Clinically, this is a vulnerable point in the lift and a time when injuries often occur. The spinal musculature remains active until the load is released and optimal erect stance is obtained.

There are two additional mechanisms which kinetically assist in lifts of heavy loads. Both mechanisms rely on the thoracodorsal fascia and its attachments for their effect. The first involves an isometric contraction of the spinal extensor muscles at the beginning of the actual lift. The second involves an isometric contraction of the abdominal muscles throughout the lift.

The erector spinae muscle is contained within an envelope of the thoracodorsal fascia which is rendered taut consequential to the broadening effect of the muscle's contraction. This action decreases the kinetic force of anterior shear at the L4 and L5 vertebrae via the midline fascial attachment to the spinous processes. More directly, the posteroanterior orientation of the lumbar iliocostalis and the lumbar longissimus muscles (see Figs 4.21, 4.22) at the L4 and L5 levels counteracts the detrimental anterior shear force when recruited isometrically.

The transversus abdominis and the internal oblique muscles facilitate the role of the thoracodorsal fascia in lifting by increasing the tension of the lateral border. When the lumbar spine is loaded in positions other than spinal flexion (i.e. between 0° and 40°), the midline ligament and the posterior ligamentous system can still be utilized to counteract anterior shear if the lateral border of the thoracodorsal fascia is rendered taut via contraction of the transversus abdominis and the internal oblique muscles.[45]

In summary, optimal and therefore safe loading and unloading of the lumbo-pelvic-hip region during activities of daily living can only occur when the myokinematics and myokinetics subserve the kinetic and kinematic requirements of the bones and joints they stabilize and move. The coordinated muscle response is dependent upon complex peripheral and central feedback mechanisms which integrate the osseous, articular and muscular function.

GAIT (Fig. 5.33)

Bipedal striding requires integrated osseous, articular and neuromuscular function of the lumbo-pelvic-hip region and is often an activity which magnifies the patient's symptoms when pathology is present. Careful observation of the gait pattern can reveal dysfunction as yet unknown to the individual. The following section will briefly outline the osteokinematic and arthrokinematic requirements of the lumbo-pelvic-hip region during one cycle of gait to illustrate the intimate biomechanical function of this region.

Efficient gait requires simultaneous osseous displacement of the femora, innominate bones, sacrum and lumbar vertebrae in all three body planes, the sagittal, coronal and transverse. Although each individual has his

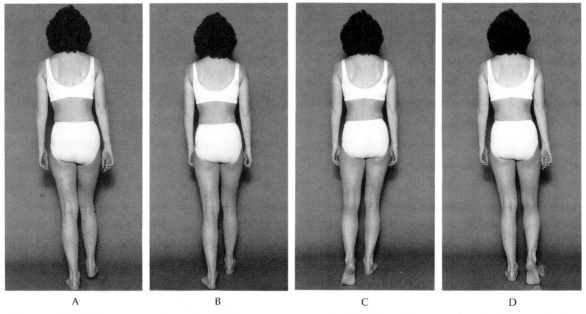

| A | B | C | D |

Fig. 5.33 Gait. This sequence shows the right leg in swing phase, heel-strike, midstance and push-off, respectively.

or her own idiosyncratic pattern of walking, the mandatory biomechanical requirements will be found in each.

Femur

From push-off through the swing phase to heel-strike, the femur moves from an extended to a flexed position. The habitual movement pattern is not a pure spin at the hip joint but rather an arcuate (impure) swing and therefore conjoined osteokinematic motions also occur. During femoral flexion, there is also adduction and lateral rotation. Arthrokinetically, the capsular ligaments of the hip joint are taken from a maximum taut position in extension, abduction and medial rotation (i.e. the close pack position) to one of relatively loose pack in flexion, adduction and lateral rotation.

From heel-strike through the midstance phase to terminal stance, the femur moves from a flexed position to an extended position. Again, this motion is not a pure spin at the hip joint but rather an arcuate or impure swing. The conjoined motions include abduction and medial rotation. Arthrokinetically, the capsular ligaments are progressively wound around the femoral neck as the body weight passes anterior to the hip joint. Through the midstance position, the winding of the capsular ligaments of the hip joint combined with the progressive osteokinetic and myokinetic forces, increases the compression of the femoral head into the acetabular fossa. Consequently, the Type III mechanoreceptors located in the ligamentum teres are fired, which reflexly facilitates the ipsilateral hip abductors necessary for stabilization of the pelvic girdle.

Restrictions of femoral mobility may be the result of either arthrokinematic or myokinematic dysfunction (stiff joint or tight muscle) and are manifested by a shortened stride length.

Pelvic girdle

From push-off through the swing phase to heel-strike, the pelvic girdle *as a unit* rotates on the femoral heads in the transverse plane towards the weight-bearing limb. The axis of this rotation is vertical between the two extremities and is dynamic rather than static. This motion decreases the amount of hip flexion/extension required for optimal stride length. Simultaneously, the pelvic girdle as a unit adducts on the weight-bearing limb, thus depressing the summit of the vertical rise of the center of gravity. As well, *intra-pelvic* torsion in the sagittal plane (see Fig. 5.17) occurs between the innominate bones and the sacrum.

Using the right extremity as an example, from push-off through the swing phase to heel-strike, the pelvic girdle as a unit rotates transversely to the left, translates anteriorly and adducts on the left femoral head. Simultaneously, the right innominate bone posteriorly rotates (flexes) and the left innominate bone anteriorly rotates (extends) driving the sacrum into right rotation. The underlying arthrokinematics for this motion at the sacroiliac joints are unknown.

Again using the right extremity, from heel-strike through midstance phase to terminal stance, the pelvic girdle as a unit rotates to the right, translates anteriorly and adducts on the right femoral head. Simultaneously, the right innominate bone anteriorly rotates (extends) and the left innominate bone posteriorly rotates (flexes) driving the sacrum into left rotation.

Kinetically, the superincumbent body weight must be transferred smoothly from one lower extremity to the other, thus necessitating optimal osseous, articular and neuromuscular function. Excessive lateral deviation of the center of gravity (lateral limp) during the midstance phase can be consequence of kinetic breakdown within the pelvic-hip complex.

Lumbar vertebrae

Osteokinematically during gait, the lower lumbar vertebrae rotate in the same sense as the sacrum. This axis about which lumbar rotation occurs is oblique (see Fig. 5.4) such that contralateral sideflexion and forward flexion occur in conjunction with the rotation.[44] The iliolumbar ligament modifies this motion at the L5–S1 segment (see Figs 5.6, 5.18, 5.19).[96] In most individuals, the total available range of motion at the lumbosacral junction is not utilized in walking and minor restrictions may not be apparent objectively, nor felt subjectively, during prolonged ambulation.

In conclusion, patients presenting with a primary lumbosacral joint dysfunction rarely complain of difficulty in walking whereas those presenting with pelvic girdle and/or hip disorders often state that walking is their most aggravating activity. It is recognized that the study of gait is incomplete without considering the influences of the foot and knee on both habitual and compensatory gait patterns at the lumbo-pelvic-hip region; however, this subject shall be left for the reader to explore once the basics are understood.

6

Wound repair and the healing process

The principles upon which the evaluation and treatment of the lumbo-pelvic-hip complex are based follow those of the body's natural healing process. Since it is doubtful that anything can be done to accelerate the normal response, the intent of therapy is to prevent and/or reverse the factors which tend to retard recovery.

Approximately three billion years ago when living organisms were unicellular, death of the cell meant death of the organism. With the evolution of multicellular organisms, so followed the process of repair after injury. Ultimately this repair process was perfected such that complete regeneration of an amputated limb was possible. Some lower vertebrates such as lizards and newts have retained this capability. The evolution of more complex life forms (e.g. the mammal) has occurred at the expense of total regenerative ability. For example, in man cardiac muscle does not regenerate after infarction, neural tissue does not regenerate after cellular death, skin does not regenerate after full-thickness injury and an amputated finger does not grow back. With few exceptions mammalian tissue responds to injury by repair rather than regeneration.

Effective treatment requires detailed knowledge of this repair process. In most tissues, repair occurs by fibrous tissue proliferation regardless of which tissue has been damaged. Although the healing process is not a state it can be divided into three phases—the substrate phase, the fibroblastic phase and

63

maturation. The physiological response of each stage dictates the appropriate therapy.

SUBSTRATE PHASE

The substrate phase (also called the lag, latent or productive phase) extends from the time of injury to the fourth to sixth day. It is characterized by the inflammatory response which prepares the wound for subsequent healing by removing the debris, necrotic tissue and bacteria. At the same time, fibroblasts migrate to the wound site. Exactly how these cells are attracted to the wound is unknown; however, several investigators[8,62,94] feel that an electric potential exists at the injury site which influences their migration. During this phase, the wound is held together by the gluing action of fibrin which has a very low breaking strength.

FIBROBLASTIC PHASE

The fibroblastic phase begins between the fourth and sixth day after injury and can last up to four to ten weeks.[94] This is the stage where therapy can dramatically effect the healing response and therefore is a critical time for treatment. At this time, the proliferating fibroblasts begin to synthesize collagen, mucopolysaccharides and glycoproteins. Regardless of the location of the wound, the fibroblasts carry on the process of wound repair by replacing the damaged structures with fibrous tissue. Tropocollagen is secreted from the fibroblasts and quickly aggregates into collagen fibers. The orientation of the fibers at this stage has been shown[8,94] to be influenced by the mechanical forces existing at the wound site. The tensile strength of the wound during the fibroblastic phase is proportional to the *quantity* of collagen present as opposed to crosslinking between the collagen fibers.[94]

MATURATION PHASE

These is no sharp demarcation between the end of the fibroblastic phase and the beginning of the maturation phase. Peacock[94] states that the quantity of collagen within the wound ceases to increase between the third and fourth week after injury. Although the collagen content within the wound remains constant or even decreases after the stage of fibroplasia, the wound continues to gain in tensile strength. This strength gain is due to two factors, intramolecular/intermolecular crosslinking of the collagen fibers and remodeling of the wound by the dissolution and reformation of the collagen fibers to give a stronger weave. The quantity of collagen is constant, it is the organization that is undergoing change. This process of remodeling may require six to twelve months for completion.

CLINICAL APPLICATION TO TREATMENT

Much of the pain and functional disability seen within the musculoskeletal system is caused by the synthesis and deposition of scar tissue and how the physical properties of collagen differ from the unwounded tissue it replaces. The therapist must therefore be aware of the ultimate function of the injured tissue, otherwise no assessment can be made of the efficacy of repair or the long-term effect. In other words, repair, while restoring structure, may seriously interfere with function. For example, the fibrous tissue which replaces ruptured muscle fibers is non-contractile, less extensible and cannot replace the function of the torn myofiber. The aim of treatment therefore, must be to control and to guide the repair process such that *optimal* structure and function are restored. Unfortunately, this is not always possible.

Can anything be done to accelerate the normal rate of healing? During the stage of fibroplasia, the tensile strength of the wound is proportional to the rate of collagen accumulation. Webster[133] has shown that ultrasound can increase the quantity of collagen synthesized, thereby increasing the tensile strength of the scar. Research[1,86] on the effects of LASER indicates that facilitation of the optimal rate of healing is possible with this modality. However, whether it is possible to shorten *the total length of time* required for maturation of the scar is controversial. What can be done, however, is to prevent the undesirable factors which tend to retard the healing process. The fibrosis can also be controlled and directed during the stages of synthesis, deposition and remodeling such that a more functional scar subserves the tissue it replaces as best it can.

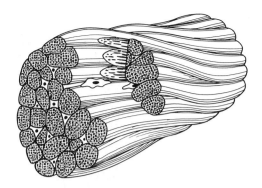

Fig. 6.2 Both tendons and ligaments are composed of a regular longitudinal arrangement of collagen fibers. (Redrawn from Warwick & Williams 1973.)[131]

Tendon

To illustrate, compare the structural characteristics of the tendon of the piriformis muscle with those of the peroneus longus muscle. The tendon of piriformis is relatively short and is not enclosed in a synovial sheath (Fig. 6.1). The collagen fibers within the tendon are oriented in a longitudinal regular manner (Fig. 6.2) consistent with the lines of stress produced when the muscle contracts. Since the Type I collagen which is present in tendon is inelastic, this arrangement allows the force generated by contraction of the muscle to be efficiently transmitted to the bony insertion on the greater trochanter. Minimal gliding of

the tendon on the adjacent structures is required for normal function.

Conversely, the tendon of the peroneus longus muscle is long and is enclosed within a synovial sheath passing beneath several fibrous tunnels on the lateral aspect of the ankle as well as within the sole of the foot (Fig. 6.3). The collagen fibers within the tendon are also oriented in a longitudinal manner (Fig. 6.2) consistent with the lines of stress produced when the muscle contracts.

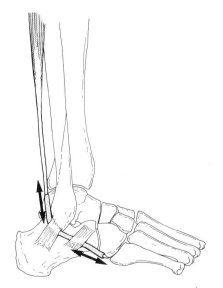

Fig. 6.3 The peroneus longus muscle, its tendon and synovial sheath.

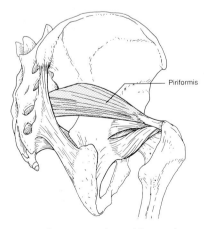

Fig. 6.1 The piriformis muscle and its tendon.

Again, this arrangement facilitates the transmission of force from the muscle belly to the bone efficiently. However, when the muscle contracts, the tendon is required to glide extensively between the adjacent structures and the restoration of this function is critical to the success of treatment.

The repair process following injury to either of these tendons is the same. The inflammatory response of the substrate phase is followed by the proliferation of fibroblasts and the production of collagen, mucopolysaccharides and glycoproteins. The orientation of the new collagen fibers at this stage of repair is influenced by mechanical deformation of the wound. Exactly how tension effects the orientation process is controversial; however, investigation[8,62] is currently focusing on the influence of the electrical field surrounding the injury site on both healing and regeneration of tissue.

In 1880, Pierre and Jacques Currie discovered that when a quartz crystal was stressed, a potential difference was produced across its faces. This was called the piezoelectric current. It is felt[8,62,94] that since collagen is crystalline in nature, a potential difference, or field of electricity, is produced when the fibers are deformed. Perhaps this deformation produces the piezoelectric current which subsequently directs the newly formed collagen fibrils. Bassett[8] has described the cellular effects of electrical current and believes these to be the trigger of wound repair. Clinically, this appears to be the most effective stage in which to implement electrical, ultrasonic, light and/or manual therapy if optimal function is to be achieved.

The tendons of the piriformis and peroneus longus muscles contain Type I collagen fibers which lie in a longitudinal direction in series with the muscle fibers. Therefore, during the fibroblastic stage of healing, treatment should be directed towards orienting the collagen fibers of both tendons longitudinally. Passive physiological mobilizations and exercise programs which *gently* stress the tendon should be started at this stage. Vigorous exercises or aggressive passive mobilizations will prevent the revascularization of the tendon and retard the healing process, so 'gentle' is the key word at this time. As well, since there is minimal intramolecular or intermolecular crosslinking of collagen fibers at this stage, strong stretching or forcing of the wound is contraindicated. More pain will definitely lead to less gain. Both ultrasound and LASER can facilitate the synthesis of collagen and are useful adjunctive modalities.

The maturation phase is the stage when things can definitely go wrong. The structure may be restored and extremely resistant to tensile forces but the function may be completely devastated. Consider the torn peroneus longus tendon in the foot. Collagen cannot differentiate between the tendon, the synovium and the fibrous tunnel. The new collagen fibers uniting the tendon will indiscriminately crosslink with those restoring the structure of the sheath or the fibrous tunnel beneath which it passes. Stability is thus restored at the expense of mobility. Since this tendon must glide extensively for normal function, a 50% reduction in the gliding ability will have profound effects on the function of the foot. By contrast, the tendon of the piriformis muscle requires little mobility between itself and the adjacent structures, and loss of this mobility will have less effect on the overall function.

There are two kinds of adhesions which can occur subsequent to the healing process, restrictive and non-restrictive. Restrictive adhesions are regularly organized with a compact arrangement of collagen fibers oriented in a longitudinal manner. Non-restrictive adhesions are randomly organized with small fiber bundles. Although the evidence is not conclusive, it is felt[94] that longitudinal slippage or friction-induced instability of collagen fibers and fibrils is the most probable method by which additional length in the scar is gained.

This information can be applied to healing tissue in the following manner. If the injured tendon is stressed repetitively during the therapeutic exercise program, an excellent environment will be created for lateral intertissue crosslinking. This facilitates tensile strength but a restrictive adhesion will also be encouraged. If, however transverse mobilizations (or frictions) of the tendon are also incorporated into the therapy session, elongation of the entire adhesion will be promoted as the collagen fibers are 'teased' apart and longitudinal slippage of the fibers occurs. The adhesion is therefore non-restrictive and both tensile strength and mobility are encouraged.

To summarize, tendon tensile strength can be effectively restored by exercise programs which apply stress to the tendon. These programs can be graduated from gentle passive stretching to vigorous eccentric loading depending upon the stage of healing. If tendon mobility is also required, attention must be directed to the lateral attachments which bind the tendon down, otherwise the stage is set for chronic repeated microtears of scar tissue such as those seen in chronic tennis elbow or chronic peroneal tendinitis following old inversion injuries of the ankle.

Ligament

Ligaments structurally resemble tendons and therefore the tensile requirements are the same. They must, however, be free to move

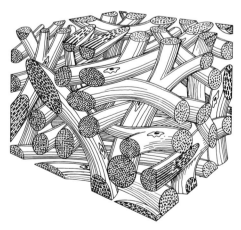

Fig. 6.4 The outer layer of the joint capsule is composed of an irregular random arrangement of collagen fibers. (Redrawn from Warwick & Williams 1973.)[131]

on the bones they cross. If a restrictive adhesion is allowed to develop, chronic repeated microtears will occur. If the adhesion can be elongated via transverse frictions, the mobility and the elasticity of the ligament will be restored. Manipulation of adhesions is a destructive treatment technique since the adhesion rarely releases where it is intended. More commonly, a fresh tear between the adhesion and normal tissue occurs which sets up another inflammatory response. If the fibroblastic phase and the maturation phase of collagen synthesis, deposition and remodeling are now treated appropriately, a new elongated adhesion will be formed which allows the necessary mobility.

Fibrous joint capsule

The structural characteristics and functional requirements of a fibrous joint capsule are quite different from those of either a tendon or ligament. The outer layer of the joint capsule is composed of an irregular random arrangement of collagen fibers (Fig. 6.4) unlike the tendon or ligament which displays a regular longitudinal arrangement (Fig. 6.2). This is a good example of function governing structure. The primary function of a ligament is to resist tensile forces between two bones, and the anatomy suits its needs ideally. The fibrous capsule, however, must be extensible to allow mobility of the joint, and since collagen is inextensible a longitudinal arrangement would inhibit mobility.

The random, irregular orientation of the collagen fibers permits mobility. When the capsule is stretched, the fibers orient themselves along the lines of tension produced by the stretch. Ultimately, the collagen fibers set the limit to the amount of extensibility permitted (Fig. 6.5). This anatomical arrangement promotes mobility while the physical characteristics of the collagen fiber itself affords end-range stability.

The repair process following capsular injury is identical to the one previously described. The initial inflammatory response is clinically apparent as traumatic arthritis. Fibroplasia and

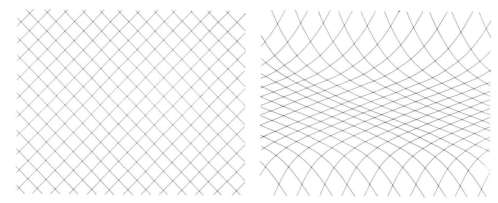

Fig. 6.5 The orientation of the collagen fibers within the joint capsule influences the degree of extensibility permitted. The random irregular orientation initially permits mobility (left). When placed under tension the reorientation of the fibers (right) ultimately restricts the motion.

collagen synthesis follows four to six days after injury. The orientation of the new fibers will not automatically assume a random arrangement if tensile forces are applied to the wound. If the patient is started on an exercise program designed to restore full range of motion, and that exercise program puts tension through the wound, longitudinal orientation of new collagen fibers will be promoted leading to increased lateral cross-linking and restricted mobility. This is not an adhesion, but rather the restoration of structure with tissue that does *not* subserve the joint capsule's function. The treatment given to any tissue is governed by the functional requirements of the damaged tissue. In this instance, both extensibility and tensile strength require restoration.

The challenge is to preserve the extensibility of the joint capsule by creating a random arrangement of small-fiber collagen bundles while simultaneously increasing the tensile strength. An extensible scar is more likely to develop if stresses are induced in a multitude of directions across the wound. Three-dimensional exercise programs, together with physiological active and passive mobilization techniques, will theoretically facilitate the random arrangement of the new collagen fibers. Unidirectional passive accessory joint

mobilizations applied for 30 seconds to 3 minutes would be counterproductive since they would stress the wound longitudinally and subsequently facilitate a longitudinal arrangement of the collagen fibers. This would actually restrict the joint mobility. It is difficult to believe, however, that even 15 minutes of passive articular mobilization could have a lasting influence on the ultimate orientation of collagen within the scar tissue since healing is a 24-hour process. Thus there is need for appropriate exercise programs and patient involvement in their own rehabilitation.

SUMMARY

Left alone, wounded tissue will repair. The efficacy of the repair process depends on how well the replacement tissue restores the tissue's original function. The role of therapy is to guide the deposition and remodeling of the scar at each stage of repair such that the resultant structure will subserve the tissue's function. To achieve this goal it is paramount that the patients become involved in their own rehabilitation program, following the principles of tissue healing, since we are all our own best healer.

7

Subjective and objective examination

Common patterns of lumbo-pelvic-hip disorders slowly emerge as clinical expertise develops in the use of consistent and repetitive subjective and objective examination. Therapists who take the time to develop disciplined examination technique will be rewarded later with the ability to recognize similar patterns of dysfunction quickly. The purpose of this section is to describe and illustrate the basic subjective and objective examination which should be part of every assesssment.

SUBJECTIVE EXAMINATION (Table 7.1)

Table 7.1 Subjective examination form

NAME:	AGE:	DR:
MODE OF ONSET:		
PAST HISTORY:	PAST TREATMENT:	
PAIN/DYSAESTHESIA: Location:	Aggravating Activities:	
	Relief Activities:	
SLEEP: Surface/Position:	Status in a.m.:	
OCCUPATION/SPORT/ HOBBIES:		
GENERAL HEALTH:	MEDICATION:	
RESULTS OF ADJUNCTIVE TESTS:		

Mode of onset

- How did the problem begin—suddenly or insidiously? With respect to wound repair, is the patient presenting during the substrate, fibroblastic or maturation phase of healing?
- Was there an element of trauma? If so, was there a major traumatic event over a short period of time, such as a fall, or was there a series of minor traumatic events over a prolonged period of time, such as the habitual use of improper lifting technique?
- Is this the first episode requiring treatment or has there been a similar past history of events? If this is a repeat episode, how long did it take to recover from the previous one and was therapy necessary at that time?

Pain/dysaesthesia

- Exactly where is the pain/dysaesthesia? Is it localized or diffuse and can its quality be described?
- How far down the limb or limbs do the symptoms radiate?
- Which activities (including how much) will aggravate the symptoms?
- What effect does prolonged sitting, standing, walking, stair-climbing and descent, rolling over in bed, getting in/out of a chair/car, cough and/or sneeze have on the pain/dysaesthesia?
- Which activities (including how much) provide relief?

Sleep

- Are the symptoms interfering with sleep? Does rest provide relief?
- What kind of bed is being slept in and what position is most frequently adopted?

Occupation/leisure activities/sport

- What level of physical activity does the patient consider their normal and essential for return to full function?
- What are the patient's goals from therapy?

The specifics of both the patient's occupation and sport are required if rehabilitation is to be successful and complete.

General information

- What is the status of the patient's general health?
- Is the patient currently taking any medication for this or any other condition?
- What are the results of any adjunctive diagnostic tests (i.e. X-ray, laboratory tests, etc.)?

OBJECTIVE EXAMINATION (Table 7.2)

Table 7.2 Objective examination form

GAIT:	POSTURE:	SAGITTAL CORONAL

HABITUAL MOVEMENT TESTS
Forward/backward bending   Standing/Sitting
   lumbar
   innominate
   sacral
Squat
Lateral bending
Striding   Right/Left
   ipsilateral kinetic test — standing
   ipsilateral kinetic test — prone

REGIONAL TESTS FOR OSSEOUS AND ARTICULAR MOBILITY/STABILITY

Lumbar spine
Positional tests (L1 to L5)
   hyperflexion
   hyperextension
Osteokinematic tests of physiological mobility (T12–L1 to L5–S1)
   flexion/extension
   sideflexion/rotation
Arthrokinematic tests of accessory joint mobility (T12–L1 to L5–S1)
   superoanterior glide
   inferoposterior glide
Arthrokinetic tests of stability
   compression
   torsion
   posteroanterior shear
   iliolumbar ligament

Pelvic girdle
Positional tests
   innominate bone
   sacrum
Osteokinematic tests of physiological mobility
   flexion/extension of the innominate bone
   flexion/extension of the sacrum
   rotation of the sacrum

Table 7.2 (cont'd)

Pelvic girdle
Arthrokinematic tests of accessory joint mobility
  anteroposterior glide
Arthrokinetic tests of stability
  transverse anterior
  transverse posterior
  superoinferior pubic symphysis
  sacrotuberous ligament

Hip
Osteokinematic tests of physiological mobility (femur)
  flexion
  extension
  abduction
  adduction
  lateral rotation
  medial rotation
  quadrant test
Arthrokinematic tests of accessory joint mobility
  distraction
  inferior glide
  posteroanterior glide
Arthrokinetic tests of stability
  proprioception
  torque test
    iliofemoral ligament
    pubofemoral ligament
    ischiofemoral ligament

MYOKINEMATIC TESTS FOR MUSCLE FUNCTION
Postural muscles   Phasic muscles

NEUROLOGICAL TESTS
Motor   Sensory   Reflex
Dural mobility

VASCULAR TESTS

SOFT TISSUE TESTS

ADJUNCTIVE TEST RESULTS

SUMMARY

Gait

Careful observation of the patient's gait pattern can be informative since normal bipedal striding requires optimal lumbo-pelvic-hip function (see Ch. 5). In particular, deviation of the center of gravity in the vertical and/or transverse planes or alteration in stride length and timing can be indicative of kinematic and/or kinetic dysfunction within the lumbo-pelvic-hip complex.

Posture

Postural asymmetry is not necessarily indica-tive of pelvic girdle dysfunction; however, pelvic girdle dysfunction is often reflected via postural asymmetry. Therefore, postural analysis in relation to the sagittal, coronal and transverse planes of the body is essential. In particular, careful observation of the distribution of body weight through the lower quadrant is required.

   Ideally, if the body is viewed from the lateral aspect, a vertical line should pass through the following points (Fig. 7.1):
1. the external auditory meatus
2. the bodies of the cervical vertebrae
3. the glenohumeral joint
4. slightly anterior to the bodies of the thoracic vertebrae, transecting the vertebrae at the thoracolumbar junction
5. the bodies of the lumbar vertebrae
6. the sacral promontory
7. slightly posterior to the coronal axis of the hip joint
8. slightly anterior to the coronal axis of the knee joint

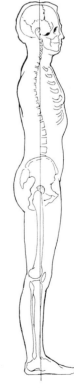

Fig. 7.1 Position of optimal postural balance in standing. (Reproduced with permission from Lee 1986.)[69]

9. slightly anterior to the talocrural joint
10. the naviculo-calcaneo-cuboid joint.

Habitual movement tests

These tests examine the habitual movement patterns of the lower quadrant; attention should be directed to both the quantity and quality of motion achieved, the patient's willingness to move as well as the presence/location of evoked symptoms. The results of these tests alone are not sufficient to diagnose local dysfunction.

Forward and backward bending

Lumbosacral junction—active physiological mobility test (flexion/extension) (Fig. 7.2). With the patient standing with his/her weight equally distributed through both lower limbs, the transverse process of the L5 vertebra is palpated bilaterally. The patient is instructed to forward/backward bend and the symmetry of motion of the transverse processes is noted. Neither rotation nor sideflexion of the L5 vertebra should occur coupled with flexion/extension during forward or backward bending (see Fig. 5.2).

Pelvic girdle—active physiological mobility tests. This is a useful preliminary test of pelvic girdle function since asymmetry of motion is present in *all* unilateral hypomobile disorders. The presence of asymmetry, however, is only indicative of lower quadrant dysfunction and is not diagnostic, and therefore the tests should be repeated in the sitting position to rule out extrinsic factors from the lower extremity (i.e. an anatomical or functional short leg). The persistence of asymmetric intra-pelvic motion during forward/backward bending while sitting should alert the examiner to intrinsic pelvic girdle dysfunction which would require further investigation.

Innominate distortion is detected in the following manner (Fig. 7.3). With the patient standing with his/her weight equally distributed through both lower limbs, the inferior aspect of the posterior superior iliac spine (PSIS) is palpated bilaterally. The patient is instructed to forward/backward bend and the

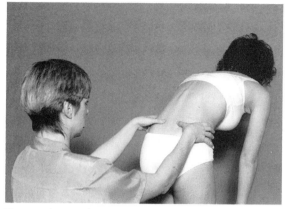

Fig. 7.2 Active physiological mobility test for flexion/extension of the lumbosacral junction. The transverse processes of the L5 vertebra should travel an equal distance in a superior direction.

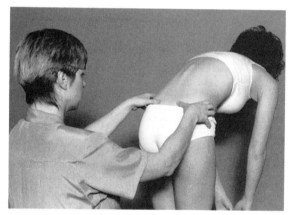

Fig. 7.3 Active physiological mobility test for forward bending of the innominate bones. The PSISs should travel an equal distance in a superior direction.

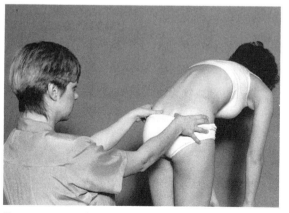

Fig. 7.4 Active physiological mobility test for forward bending of the sacrum. The ILAs of the sacrum should travel an equal distance in a superior direction without deviating in the anteroposterior plane.

symmetry of motion of the PSISs is noted.

Sacral distortion is detected by repeating the test while palpating the sacral base or the inferior lateral angle (ILA) bilaterally (Fig. 7.4).

Hip—active physiological mobility test (weight-bearing flexion). The ability of the hip joint to obtain and to bear full weight in flexion is tested by asking the patient to perform a bilateral and/or unilateral squat.

Lateral bending—active physiological mobility test

With the patient standing with his/her weight equally distributed through both lower limbs, he/she is instructed to sidebend to alternate sides (see Fig. 5.16). The ability of the pelvic girdle to translate laterally to the opposite side without deviation is noted (see Ch. 5 for the specific regional osteokinematics required during this test).

Striding[97]—active physiological mobility tests (intra-pelvic torsion)

The following tests examine intra-pelvic torsion of the lumbo-pelvic-hip complex (see Fig. 5.17), the essential biomechanical component of all movement other than forward/backward bending of the trunk.

Ipsilateral kinetic test (standing) for innominate flexion/lateral rotation, and sacral rotation (Fig. 7.5).[37,69,71] With the patient standing with his/her weight evenly distributed through both lower limbs, the inferior aspect of the PSIS is palpated with one thumb while the other palpates the median sacral crest directly parallel. The patient is instructed to flex the ipsilateral femur at the hip joint and the inferomedial displacement of the PSIS relative to the sacrum is noted.

Attention should also be directed to the patient's ability to transfer weight through the contralateral limb and to maintain balance. Intra-pelvic kinetic dysfunction is often manifested at this point. The test is then repeated on and compared to the opposite side.

If the right innominate bone is used as an example, the right ipsilateral kinetic test examines the ability of the right innominate bone to flex/laterally rotate (posteriorly rotate) while not weight-bearing, the sacrum to right rotate and the L5 vertebra to right rotate (see Figs 5.17, 5.18). The left ipsilateral kinetic test examines the ability of the left innominate bone to flex/laterally rotate while not weight-bearing, the sacrum to left rotate and the L5 vertebra to left rotate (see Fig. 5.19). A third test is required to examine the ability of the innominate bone to extend/medially rotate (anteriorly rotate).

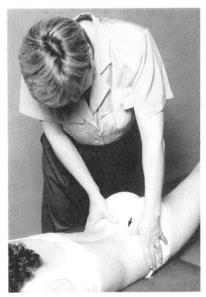

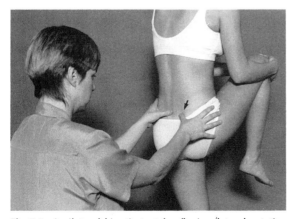

Fig. 7.5 Ipsilateral kinetic test for flexion/lateral rotation of the innominate bone and sacral rotation. Note the inferomedial displacement of the PSIS (arrow).

Fig. 7.6 Ipsilateral kinetic test for extension/medial rotation of the innominate bone and sacral rotation. Note the superolateral displacement of the PSIS (arrow).

Ipsilateral kinetic test (prone lying) for innominate extension/medial rotation, and sacral rotation (Fig. 7.6).[97] With the patient prone, the PSIS of the innominate bone is palpated with one thumb while the other palpates the median sacral crest directly parallel. The patient is instructed to extend the ipsilateral femur at the hip joint and the superolateral displacement of the PSIS relative to the sacrum is noted. The test is repeated on and compared to the opposite side.

Regional tests for osseous and articular mobility/stability

Lumbosacral junction—positional tests

When interpreting the mobility findings, the position of the joint (positional testing) at the beginning of the test should be correlated with the subsequent mobility noted, since alterations in joint mobility may merely be a reflection of an altered starting position. To determine the position of the restricted L5 vertebra, the posteroanterior relationship between the transverse processes of the L5 vertebra and the sacral base is noted in hyperflexion and hyperextension. The influence of

muscular hypertrophy and atrophy should be considered when interpreting the positional findings.

Hyperflexion (Fig. 7.7). With the patient sitting, feet supported and the lumbar spine fully flexed, the transverse processes of the L5 vertebra are palpated with the thumbs. The posteroanterior relationship of the transverse processes of the L5 vertebra relative to the sacral base is noted. A posterior right transverse process of the L5 vertebra relative to the sacral base is indicative of a right rotated position of the L5–S1 joint complex in hyperflexion.

Hyperextension (Fig. 7.8). With the patient prone and the lumbar spine fully extended, the transverse processes of the L5 vertebra are palpated with the thumbs. The posteroanterior relationship of the transverse processes of the L5 vertebra relative to the sacral base is noted. A posterior right transverse process of the L5 vertebra relative to the sacral base is indicative of a right rotated position of the L5–S1 joint complex in hyperextension.

Lumbosacral junction—osteokinematic tests of physiological mobility

Flexion/extension (Fig. 7.9). With the patient sidelying, hips and knees flexed and supported on the therapist's abdomen, the

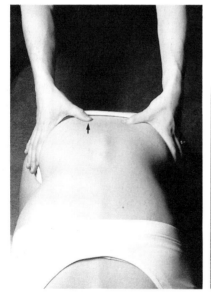
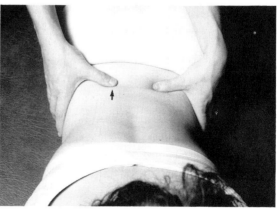

Figs 7.7 and 7.8 Positional testing of the lumbosacral junction in hyperflexion (Fig. 7.7) and in hyperextension (Fig. 7.8). Note the relative posterior position of the therapist's right thumb (arrow) when compared to the left.

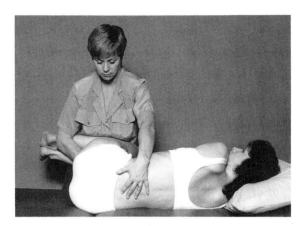

Fig. 7.9 Test for passive flexion/extension of the lumbosacral junction.

interspinous space between the L5 vertebra and the sacrum is palpated with the cranial hand. The caudal arm and hand supports the patient's legs above the ankles. The lumbosacral junction is passively flexed/extended and the quantity and quality of motion are noted.

Sideflexion/rotation (Fig. 7.10). With the patient sidelying, hips and knees slightly flexed, the interspinous space between the L5 vertebra and the sacrum is palpated with the cranial hand. The caudal arm and hand palpates the pelvic girdle in an obliquely distolateral direction. The lumbosacral junction is passively sideflexed/rotated about the appropriate oblique axis and the quantity and quality of motion are noted.

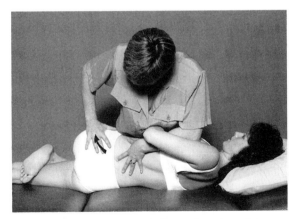

Fig. 7.10 Test for passive sideflexion/rotation of the lumbosacral junction. Note the obliquity of the motion required (arrow).

Lumbosacral junction—arthrokinematic tests of accessory joint mobility

Superoanterior glide (Fig. 7.11). With the patient sitting, feet supported and the lumbar spine fully flexed, the transverse process of the L5 vertebra is palpated unilaterally with the thumbs. A superoanterior pressure is applied in varying directions and the quantity and end feel of motion are noted and compared to the opposide side as well as to the L4–L5 joint complex. The findings are correlated with the positional findings previously recorded.

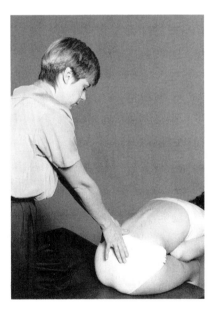

Fig. 7.11 Test for passive accessory superoanterior glide at the lumbosacral junction.

Inferoposterior glide (Fig. 7.12) With the patient prone and the lumbar spine fully extended, the transverse process of the L5 vertebra is palpated unilaterally with the thumbs. An inferior pressure is applied in varying directions and the quantity and end feel of motion are noted and compared to the opposite side as well as to the L4–L5 joint complex. The findings are correlated with the positional findings previously recorded.

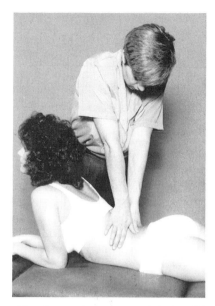

Fig. 7.12 Test for passive accessory inferior glide at the lumbosacral junction.

Lumbosacral junction—arthrokinetic tests of stability

Compression (Fig. 7.13). With the patient lying supine and the hips and knees fully

flexed, the lower extremities are cradled. Compression is applied to the vertebral column by applying a cranial force parallel to the table through the flexed lower extremities. The quantity of motion, the end feel and the presence of pain are noted.

Torsion (Fig. 7.14). With the patient lying prone, the spinous process of the L5 vertebra is palpated with the cranial thumb. With the caudal hand, the anterior aspect of the contralateral innominate bone is grasped. Segmental torsion is applied by rotating the pelvis *unphysiologically* about a pure vertical axis beneath the fixed L5 vertebra (see Fig. 5.9). The joint reaction to this stress is noted both objectively (i.e. reactive muscle spasm) as well as subjectively. This test also stresses the iliolumbar ligament and the ventral sacroiliac ligament, and therefore the location of pain is critical to kinetic analysis.

Posteroanterior shear (Fig. 7.15). With the patient lying prone, the spinous process of the L5 vertebra is palpated with the heel of the hand. The palpating hand may be reinforced by the other for additional force. A slow, steady, posteroanterior shear is applied to the

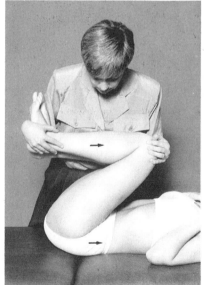
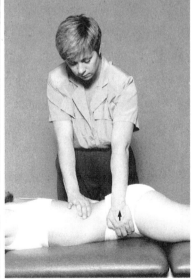
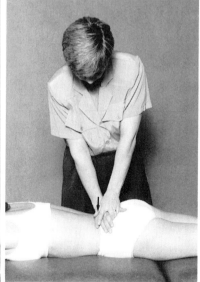

Fig. 7.13   Fig. 7.14   Fig. 7.15

Figs 7.13, 7.14 and 7.15 Arthrokinetic tests. Compression stress test (Fig. 7.13). Torsion stress test (Fig. 7.14). Note that the rotation induced at the lumbosacral junction is about a pure vertical axis and is therefore unphysiological. Posteroanterior shear stress test (Fig. 7.15) for arthrokinetic stability of the lumbosacral junction.

L5 vertebra. The quantity of motion as well as the joint reaction to this applied stress (i.e. reactive muscle spasm) is noted.

Iliolumbar ligament. With the patient in sidelying, the lower arm positioned behind the back and the upper arm hanging over the edge of the table, the interspinous space between the L5 vertebra and the sacrum is palpated with the cranial hand. The lumbosacral junction is rotated to the limit of the range of motion. From this position, the posterior band of the iliolumbar ligament is stressed as follows. With the caudal hand, the lower extremities are supported bilaterally, the hips and knees comfortably flexed and supported on the therapist's abdomen. A slow, steady, posterior force is applied to the pelvic girdle and maintained for 20 seconds. The provocation of local pain is noted. With the lumbosacral junction still rotated to the limit of the range of motion, the anterior and superior bands are stressed as follows. The hips and knees are comfortably flexed and allowed to rest on the table. With the caudal hand, the uppermost innominate bone is palpated in a distolateral direction. A slow, steady inferior force is applied to the pelvic girdle and maintained for 20 seconds. The provocation of local symptoms is noted.

Pelvic girdle—positional tests

When interpreting the mobility findings, the position of the bone (positional testing) at the beginning of the test should be correlated with the subsequent mobility, since alterations in joint mobility may merely be a reflection of an altered starting position.

Innominate bone (Figs 7.16, 7.17). To determine the position of the restricted innominate bone relative to its counterpart, the superoinferior/mediolateral relationship of the anterior superior iliac spines, the posterior superior iliac spines and the ischial tuberosities is noted with the vertebral column in a neutral position (i.e. patient is supine/prone). As well, the tension of the sacrotuberous ligament at its inferomedial border is assessed and correlated with the positional findings of the bones

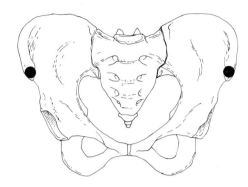

Fig. 7.16 Points of anterior palpation for positional testing of the innominate bone.

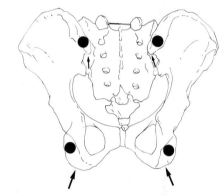

Fig. 7.17 Points of posterior palpation (large arrows) for positional testing of the innominate bone. The inferior aspect (small arrows) of the PSIS and the ischial tuberosity (dots) are palpated bilaterally and the superoinferior/mediolateral relationship noted.

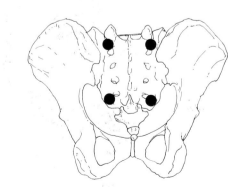

Fig. 7.18 Points of palpation for positional testing of the sacrum.

it attaches to. For example, if the innominate bone is flexed (posteriorly rotated), the sacrotuberous ligament should be taut since the points of attachment are attenuated. However, if the innominate bone is extended (anteriorly rotated), the sacrotuberous ligament should be relatively slack since the points of attachment are approximated.

Sacrum (Fig. 7.18). Positional testing of the sacrum between the innominate bones should be evaluated in all three positions of the trunk—hyperflexion, hyperextension and neutral. The sacral position is initially assessed in hyperflexion with the patient sitting, feet supported and the lumbar spine fully flexed, subsequently in neutral (prone) and finally in hyperextension with the patient prone and the lumbar spine fully extended. To determine the position of the sacrum, a comparison is made of the posteroanterior relationship of the inferior lateral angles, the posteroanterior relationship of the sacral base and the depth of the two sacral sulci. An anterior right sacral base, a deep right sacral sulcus together with a posterior left inferior lateral angle is indica-

tive of a left rotated sacrum. An anterior left sacral base, a deep left sacral sulcus together with a posterior right inferior lateral angle is indicative of a right rotated sacrum. An anterior left sacral base, a deep left sacral sulcus together with a posterior left inferior lateral angle is indicative of a unilateral left sacral flexion. These positional findings may only be manifested in one position of the vertebral column (i.e. hyperflexion), and it is therefore necessary to evaluate in all three.

Pelvic girdle—osteokinematic tests of physiological mobility

Flexion/extension (posterior/anterior rotation) of the innominate bone (Fig. 7.19). With the patient sidelying, hips and knees comfortably flexed, the anterior aspect of the iliac crest of the uppermost innominate bone is palpated with one hand while the other palpates the ipsilateral ischial tuberosity. The innominate bone is passively flexed and extended (posteriorly and anteriorly rotated) on the sacrum and the quantity of motion is

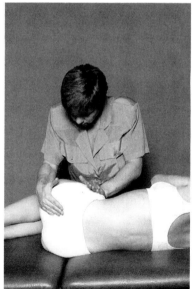 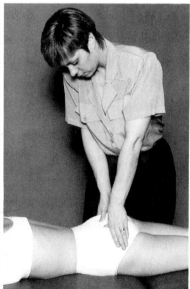 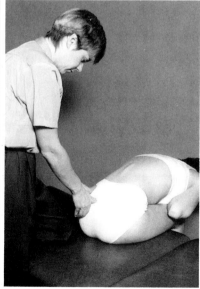

Fig. 7.19   **Fig. 7.20**   **Fig. 7.21**

Fig. 7.19 Test for passive flexion/extension (posterior/anterior rotation) of the innominate bone.
Fig. 7.20 Test for passive extension of the sacrum in neutral.
Fig. 7.21 Test for passive rotation of the sacrum.

noted and correlated with the positional findings previously recorded.

Flexion/extension of the sacrum (Fig. 7.20). Mobility testing of the sacrum should be evaluated in all three positions of the trunk—hyperflexion, neutral and hyperextension—especially if positional asymmetry has been observed.

With the patient sitting, feet supported and the lumbar spine fully flexed, the sacral base and then the inferior lateral angle are palpated bilaterally. A posteroanterior pressure is applied in variable directions until the plane of the sacroiliac joint is located (see Ch. 4). The quantity of motion is noted and correlated with the positional findings previously recorded. The test is repeated with the sacrum in neutral and then in hyperextension.

Rotation of the sacrum (Fig. 7.21). With the patient sitting, feet supported and the lumbar spine fully flexed, the sacral base and then the inferior lateral angle is palpated unilaterally. A posteroanterior pressure is applied in variable directions until the plane of the sacroiliac joint is located (see Ch. 4). The quantity of motion is noted and correlated with the positional findings previously recorded. The test is repeated with the sacrum in neutral and then in hyperextension.

Pelvis girdle—arthrokinematic tests of accessory joint mobility

The underlying arthrokinematics of the sacroiliac joint and the pubic symphysis which fulfil the osteokinematic function of the innominate bones and the sacrum are at best theorectical (see Ch. 5). Investigators[9,81] have recently proposed that deformation of the articular fibrocartilage is responsible for the observed motion rather than specific 'swings, spins and glides' of the articular surfaces. Accessory mobility testing of the sacroiliac joint can only be adjunctive given the biomechanical uncertainty.

Anteroposterior glide. With the patient lying supine, the sacral base is palpated with the fingertips of the cranial hand. The anterior aspect of the iliac crest and the ASIS is palpated with the caudal hand. An anteroposterior glide of the innominate bone is applied in varying directions and the quantity and end feel of motion are noted and compared to the opposite side.

Pelvic girdle—arthrokinetic tests of stability

Transverse anterior stress test (Fig. 7.22). With the patient lying supine, the medial aspect of the anterior superior iliac spine is palpated bilaterally with the heels of the crossed hands. A slow, steady, posterolateral force is applied through the pelvic girdle, thus stressing the ventral sacroiliac ligaments and the transverse pubic ligament. The force is maintained for 20 seconds and the provocation of local pain is noted. The ventral sacroiliac ligament can be palpated at Baer's point located approximately one inch medial to the ASIS deep within the pelvic bowl. Exquisite tenderness at this point is indicative of either an irritable ligament and/or iliacus muscle spasm.

Transverse posterior stress test (Fig. 7.23). With the patient sidelying, hips and knees comfortably flexed, the anterolateral aspect of

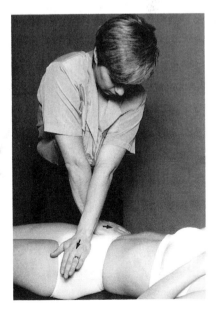

Fig. 7.22 Transverse anterior stress test for arthrokinetic stability of the pelvic girdle.

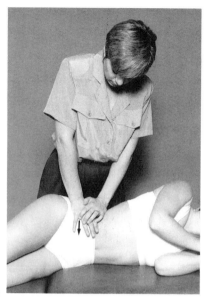

Fig. 7.23 Transverse posterior stress test for arthrokinetic stability of the pelvic girdle.

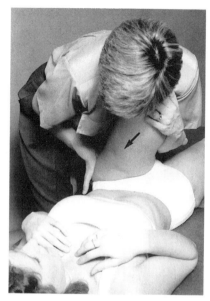

Fig. 7.25 Sacrotuberous ligament stress test.

the uppermost iliac crest is palpated. A slow, steady, medial force is applied through the pelvic girdle, thus stressing the dorsal sacroiliac ligaments. The force is maintained for 20 seconds and the provocation of local pain is noted.

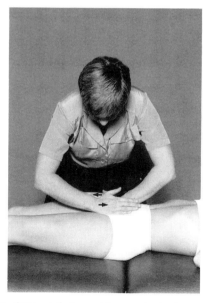

Fig. 7.24 Superoinferior pubic symphysis stress test for arthrokinetic stability of the pelvic girdle.

Superoinferior pubic symphysis stress test (Fig. 7.24). With the patient lying supine, the superior pubic rami are palpated with the heels of the hands. A slow, steady, superoinferior shear force is applied to the pubic symphysis and the provocation of local pain is noted.

Sacrotuberous ligament stress test (Fig. 7.25). With the patient lying supine and the ipsilateral hip flexed and adducted, the top of the flexed knee is palpated. The other hand palpates the sacrotuberous ligament. The innominate bone is flexed/medially rotated until tension of the sacrotuberous ligament is perceived. From this position, a slow, steady, longitudinal force is applied through the femur in an obliquely lateral direction to further stress the ligament. The force is maintained for 20 seconds and the provocation of local pain is noted.

Hip—osteokinematic tests of physiological mobility

Flexion (Fig. 7.26). With the patient lying supine, the flexed knee of the lower extremity to be tested is palpated with the caudal hand. The anterior aspect of the iliac crest and the

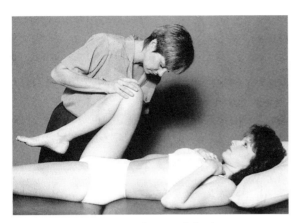

Fig. 7.26 Test for passive flexion of the femur.

anterior superior iliac spine are palpated with the cranial hand. The femur is passively flexed at the hip joint until flexion of the ipsilateral innominate bone begins. At that point, the limit of available range for femoral flexion has occurred. Both the quantity of femoral flexion as well as the end feel of motion are noted. The test is repeated on and compared to the opposite extremity.

Extension (Fig. 7.27). With the patient supine, lying at the end of the table, one femur is fully flexed against the trunk, held by the patient and supported against the thera-

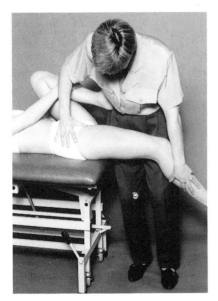

Fig. 7.27 Test for passive extension of the femur.

pist's lateral thorax. The anterior aspect of the iliac crest and the anterior superior iliac spine of the limb being tested are palpated with the cranial hand. With the caudal hand, the therapist guides the femur into extension until extension of the ipsilateral innominate bone begins. At that point, the limit of available range for femoral extension has occurred. Both the quantity of femoral extension as well as the end feel of motion are noted. The test is repeated on and compared to the opposite extremity.

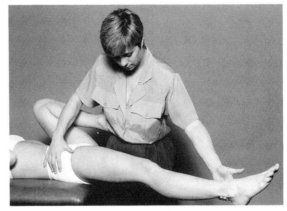

Fig. 7.28 Test for passive abduction of the femur.

Abduction/adduction (Fig. 7.28). With the patient supine, lying at the end of the table, one femur is fully flexed against the trunk, held by the patient and supported against the therapist's lateral thorax. The anterior aspect of the iliac crest and the anterior superior iliac spine of the limb being tested are palpated with the cranial hand. With the caudal hand, the therapist guides the femur into abduction/adduction until lateral bending of the pelvic girdle beneath the vertebral column begins. At that point, the limit of femoral abduction/adduction has been reached. Both the quantity of femoral abduction/adduction as well as the end feel of motion are noted. The test is repeated on and compared to the opposite extremity.

Lateral/medial rotation (Fig. 7.29). With the patient lying supine, the lower extremity to be tested is palpated above the ankle with the

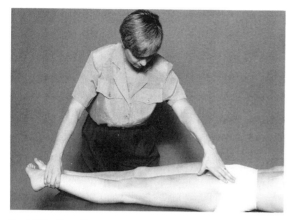

Fig. 7.29 Test for passive medial rotation of the femur in neutral.

caudal hand. The test can be performed in varying degrees of hip flexion/extension to assist in the differentiation between an articular and myofascial restriction. The anterior aspect of the iliac crest and the anterior superior iliac spine are palpated with the cranial hand. The femur is passively laterally/ medially rotated until rotation of the innominate bone begins. At that point, the limit of available range for femoral rotation has occurred. Both the quantity of femoral rotation as well as the end feel of motion are

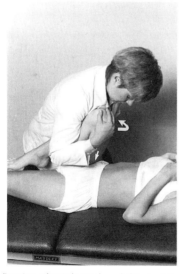

Fig. 7.30 Passive physiological mobility test (quadrant test) of the hip joint.

noted. The test is repeated on and compared to the opposite extremity.

Quadrant test (Fig. 7.30). With the patient lying supine, the flexed knee of the lower extremity to be tested is palpated with the caudal hand. The anterior aspect of the iliac crest and the anterior superior iliac spine are palpated with the cranial hand. The femur is passively flexed, adducted, medially rotated and longitudinally compressed to scour the inner aspect of the joint. From this position, the femur is taken into abduction and lateral rotation while maintaining the degree of femoral flexion and longitudinal compression. Both the quality of motion and the presence/location of pain are noted. The test is repeated on and compared to the opposite extremity.

Hip—arthrokinematic tests of accessory joint mobility

The arthrokinematics of the hip joint are relatively limited in comparison to the gross physiological movements they facilitate. Consequently, movement analysis based solely on the quantity of arthrokinematic motion (swing or glide) will often be inadequate. At the hip joint, particular attention should be paid to the quality and the end feel of osteokinematic motion for differentiation between restrictions of articular and myofascial etiology.

Distraction (Fig. 7.31). With the patient lying supine and the femur flexed to 30° (resting position of the hip joint), the proximal thigh is palpated. The joint is distracted by applying a distolateral force parallel to the neck of the femur. The posteroanterior orientation of the applied force will vary depending upon the degree of femoral anteversion present. The quantity of motion, the end feel and the presence/location of pain are noted.

Inferior glide (Fig. 7.32). With the patient lying supine and the femur flexed to 30°, the proximal thigh is palpated. An inferior femoral glide is induced by applying a inferolateral force along the longitudinal axis of the femur. The quantity of motion, the end feel and the

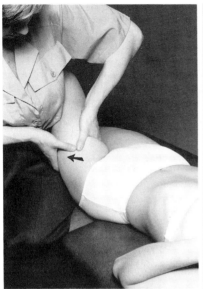
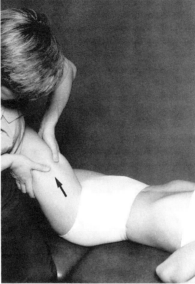
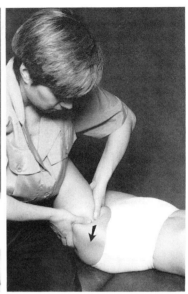

Fig. 7.31   Fig. 7.32   Fig. 7.33

Figs 7.31, 7.32 and 7.33 Arthrokinematic tests at the hip: for distraction, for passive accessory inferior glide, and for passive accessory posteroanterior glide.

presence/location of pain are noted.

Posteroanterior glide (Fig. 7.33). With the patient lying supine and the femur flexed to 30°, the proximal thigh is palpated. A postero-anterior glide is induced by applying a posterolateral/anteromedial force parallel to the plane of the acetabular fossa. The quantity of motion, the end feel and the presence/location of pain are noted.

Hip—arthrokinetic tests of stability

Proprioception/arthrokinetic stability (Fig. 7.34). This is a useful preliminary test of inte-grated neuromuscular function (see Ch. 4—Microscopic articular neurology) of the weight-bearing hip joint. With the patient standing in front of a plumb-line, he/she is instructed to bear weight unilaterally without support and to subsequently close the eyes. The degree of lateral shift of the center of gravity from the plumb-line is observed and compared to the opposite side.

Torque test (Fig. 7.35). This is a global test of passive arthrokinetic stability for the hip joint. The intent is to stress all of the capsular liga-ments synonymously. If the test is painless,

then the following tests are not required. If, however, the test reproduces local pain, then subsequent differentiation is required.

With the patient supine, lying close to the

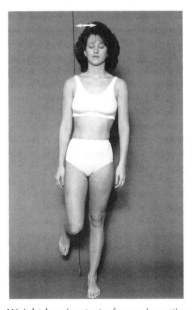

Fig. 7.34 Weight-bearing test of proprioception and arthrokinetic stability at the hip. Note the degree of lateral shift of the center of gravity from the plumb-line (arrow).

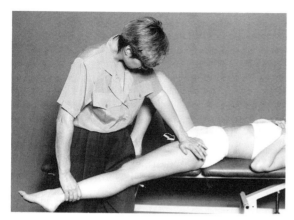

Fig. 7.35 Torque test of arthrokinetic stability at the hip joint.

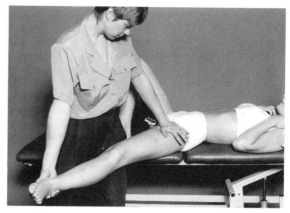

Fig. 7.36 Pubofemoral ligament stress test.

edge of the table, the ipsilateral femur is extended (over the edge) until extension of the innominate bone begins. The femur is then medially rotated to the limit of the physiological range of motion. The proximal thigh is palpated and a slow, steady, postero-lateral force is applied along the line of the neck of the femur to further stress the capsular ligaments via distraction. The force is maintained for 20 seconds and the provo-cation of local pain is noted.

Inferior band of the iliofemoral ligament. This ligament is under the greatest tension when the femur is fully extended. If passive femoral extension elicits the greatest amount of pain, this ligament may be the etiological factor.

Iliotrochanteric band of the iliofemoral liga-ment. With the patient supine, lying close to the edge of the table, the ipsilateral femur is slightly extended, *adducted* and fully laterally rotated. The distal femur is fixed against the therapist's thigh and the proximal femur is palpated. A slow, steady, posterolateral force is applied along the line of the neck of the femur and the provocation of local pain is noted.

Pubofemoral ligament (Fig. 7.36). With the patient lying supine, the ipsilateral femur is slightly extended, *abducted* and fully laterally rotated. The distal femur is fixed against the therapist's thigh and the proximal femur is palpated. A slow, steady, posterolateral force

is applied along the line of the neck of the femur and the provocation of local pain is noted.

Ischiofemoral ligament. With the patient lying supine, the ipsilateral femur is slightly extended, abducted and fully *medially* rotated. The distal femur is fixed against the therapist's thigh and the proximal femur is palpated. A slow, steady, anterolateral force is applied along the line of the neck of the femur and the provocation of local pain is noted.

Myokinematic tests for muscle function

If the regional tests of osseous/articular mobility fail to reveal the etiology of dysfunc-tion, the following tests of myokinematic function may assist in determining the cause. Relative to the pelvic girdle, the postural muscles which tend to tighten[56,57,58] should be assessed for their extensibility and influence on the mobility of the lumbo-pelvic-hip complex. The postural muscles include:
1. erector spinae/quadratus lumborum
2. hamstrings
3. rectus femoris
4. iliopsoas
5. tensor fascia lata
6. adductors
7. piriformis.

Erector spinae/quadratus lumborum

With the patient sitting, feet supported and

the vertebral column in a neutral position, he/she is instructed to forward bend. The quantity of the available motion, the symmetry/asymmetry of the paravertebral muscles and the presence/absence of a multisegmental spinal curve at the limit of range are noted. A multisegmental rotoscoliosis may be indicative of unilateral tightness of the erector spinae and/or quadratus lumborum muscles.

Hamstrings (semimembranosus, semitendinosus, biceps femoris)

With the patient lying supine, the lower extremity to be tested is palpated above the ankle. While maintaining the knee in extension, the femur is flexed at the hip joint. The therapist's cranial hand monitors any subsequent flexion of the innominate bone via the anterior aspect of the iliac crest and the anterior superior iliac spine. The extensibility of the hamstring muscle group has been reached when the innominate bone is felt to flex (posteriorly rotate). Although further femoral flexion is possible, it is secondary to

flexion of the innominate bone. Both the quantity and the end feel of motion are noted. The test is repeated on and compared to the opposite extremity.

Iliopsoas, rectus femoris, anterior band of tensor fascia lata (Figs 7.37, 7.38, 7.39)

With the patient supine, lying at the end of the table, one femur is fully flexed against the trunk, held by the patient and supported against the therapist's lateral thorax. The anterior aspect of the iliac crest and the anterior superior iliac spine of the limb being tested are palpated with the cranial hand. With the caudal hand, the therapist guides the femur into extension with the knee extended to test the length of the iliopsoas muscle and then with the knee flexed to test the length of the rectus femoris muscle. Both the quantity of femoral extension and knee flexion as well as the end feel of motion are noted. The test is repeated on and compared to the opposite extremity.

An inextensible iliopsoas muscle will restrict extension of the femur regardless of the

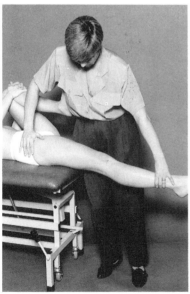 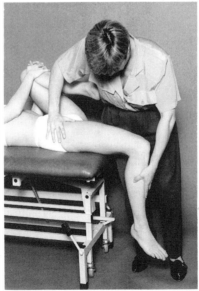 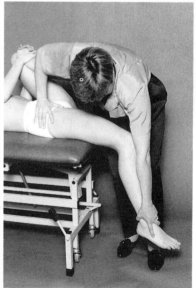

Fig. 7.37 **Fig. 7.38** **Fig. 7.39**

Figs 7.37, 7.38 and 7.39 Tests for extensibility of the iliopsoas muscle, the rectus femoris muscle and the anterior band of the tensor fascia lata muscle.

position of the knee whereas an inextensible rectus femoris muscle will only restrict extension of the femur if the knee is flexed.

If the anterior band of the tensor fascia lata muscle is tight, full femoral extension and knee flexion will occur; however, knee flexion will only be possible in conjunction with lateral tibial rotation. If the tibial rotation is passively blocked during the test, knee flexion will be restricted.

Middle band of tensor fascia lata (Fig. 7.40)

With the patient sidelying, the bottom limb comfortably flexed, the anteromedial aspect of the femur is grasped with the caudal hand and the flexed knee supported by the therapist's caudal hand and forearm. The pelvic girdle is supported with the cranial hand while the caudal hand flexes, abducts and then extends the femur in one smooth motion. The femur is then guided into adduction while the knee is maintained in flexion. Both the quantity of femoral adduction and the quality of the end feel are noted. The test is repeated on and compared to the opposite extremity. An inextensible tensor fascia lata muscle will restrict femoral adduction during this test.

Adductors

With the patient supine, lying at the end of the table, one femur is fully flexed against the trunk, held by the patient and supported against the therapist's lateral thorax. The anterior aspect of the iliac crest and the anterior superior iliac spine of the limb being tested are palpated with the cranial hand. With the caudal hand, the therapist guides the femur into abduction. Both the quantity of femoral abduction as well as the end feel of motion are noted. The test is repeated on and compared to the opposite extremity.

Piriformis (Fig. 7.41)

With the patient lying supine, the lower extremity is grasped at the flexed knee. The lateral aspect of the iliac crest and the anterior superior iliac spine are palpated with the cranial hand, while the caudal hand flexes the femur to 60° of flexion. At this point, the piriformis muscle acts as a pure abductor of the femur.[60] Before 60° it also laterally rotates the femur, while after 60° it medially rotates the femur.[60] From 60° of femoral flexion, the

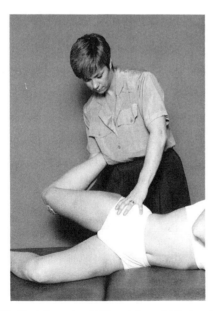

Fig. 7.40 Test for extensibility of the middle band of the tensor fascia lata muscle (Ober's test).

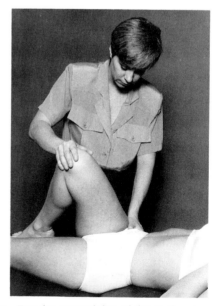

Fig. 7.41 Test for extensibility of the piriformis muscle. At 60° of femoral flexion, this muscle acts as a pure femoral abductor.

femur is guided into adduction with the caudal hand while the cranial hand monitors the subsequent medial rotation (inflaring) of the innominate bone. The extensibility of the piriformis muscle has been reached when the innominate bone is felt to medially rotate, and although further adduction of the femur is possible it is secondary to the medial rotation of the innominate bone. If the femur is taken beyond 60° of flexion, lateral femoral rotation is required to fully stretch the muscle. Both the quantity and the end feel of motion are noted. The test is repeated on and compared to the opposite extremity.

Myokinematic testing is completed with a detailed examination of the contractile tissue function of all the muscles attaching to the lumbo-pelvic-hip complex. The presence and the location of pain evoked during resisted testing is correlated with the muscle's strength, thus enabling the therapist to reach a diagnosis of muscle 'sprain' and/or rupture. Grades 1 and 2 muscle sprains are painfully strong when resisted isometrically as opposed to Grade 3 sprains (i.e. complete ruptures) which are relatively painfree and weak when resisted isometrically. Of course, there exists an entire spectrum of dysfunction between the two extremes.

Relative to the pelvic girdle, the phasic muscles which tend to weaken (i.e. the abdominals; gluteus maximus, medius and minimus; vastus lateralis, medialis and inter-medius) should be specifically assessed for strength.[56,57,58] The tests for evaluating muscle strength should be familiar to all clinicians and need not be described here.

Neurological tests

These tests examine the conductivity of the motor and sensory nerves relative to the lumbosacral plexus as well as the mobility of the dura through the intervertebral foramina.

Motor tests

The L2 to S2 motor nerve roots are evaluated clinically via the peripheral muscles they

innervate. Although there are no true peripheral myotomes in the lower quadrant (one muscle solely innervated by one nerve root), specific muscles known as *key muscles* are primarily innervated by one motor nerve and their function is a reflection of the neurological innervation. Initially, a maximal contraction is elicited from the key muscle and the quantity and quality of strength are compared to the opposite side. If the muscle tests are strong, six submaximal contractions are elicited to detect accelerated fatiguability—a common finding of neurological impedance.

The motor nerves and the key muscles which are evaluated include:
L2 — iliopsoas, adductors
L3 — adductors, quadriceps
L4 — quadriceps, tibialus anterior
L5 — extensor hallucis, extensor digitorum, peronei
S1 — hamstrings, gastrocnemius
S2 — hamstrings, gluteus maximus.

Sensory tests

The L1 to S2 sensory nerve roots are evaluated clinically via the dermatomes they innervate. Dermatome maps can be confusing since variations in dermatome distribution exist from individual to individual. As well, impedance of sensory conductivity may be reflected in a variety of dysaesthesia ranging from slight hyperaesthesia to complete anaesthesia. Detailed examination of the distal extent of the dermatome is useful in detecting early neurological interference. One of the first signs of sensory dysfunction is hyperaesthesia within a specific dermatome. This sign tends to occur long before sensation becomes reduced or obliterated completely and its existence is often a surprise to the patient.

Although individual variability is recognized, the following description of dermatome distribution is one commonly seen:
L1 — upper posterior buttock, anterior groin
L2 — middle posterior buttock, anterior thigh to the knee

L3 — lower posterior buttock, anterior thigh to the medial knee and occasionally distal to the medial malleolus

L4 — lateral thigh, medial leg, dorsum of the foot to the great toe

L5 — lateral leg, dorsum of the foot to toes 2, 3, 4, sole of the foot (excluding the heel) to toes 1, 2, 3

S1 — posterior thigh, leg, lateral border of the foot to dorsum and sole, to toes 4 and 5

S2 — posterior thigh, leg to heel

S3, S4 — perineal region.

Reflex tests

The spinal reflexes are evaluated via the myotatic response to stretch of the key muscle innervated by the root in question. They include the following:

L3, L4 — quadriceps (i.e. knee jerk)

L5, S1, S2 — gastrocnemius (i.e. ankle jerk).

The integrity of the spinal cord is evaluated by the plantar response test.

Dural mobility tests

The mobility of the dura mater surrounding the L2 to S2 nerve roots is evaluated by two tests, the femoral nerve stretch test and the straight leg raise test.

Femoral nerve stretch test. With the patient prone, the lower extremity is palpated above the ankle. The lower leg is passively flexed at the knee joint and the quantity and end feel of motion are noted. When the mobility of the dura mater of the L2, L3 and/or L4 nerve roots is restricted, hip extension and knee flexion are restricted by pain felt posteriorly in the lumbar spine.

Straight leg raise test. With the patient lying supine, the lower extremity is palpated above the ankle. While maintaining the knee in extension and the femur in slight adduction/medial rotation, the femur is flexed at the hip joint. The quantity and end feel of motion are noted. When the mobility of the dura mater of the L4, L5, S1, and/or S2 nerve roots is restricted, hip flexion is limited to 30° to 60° by both pain and muscle spasm.

Vascular tests

These tests screen the circulatory status of the lower extremity. Careful observation of the skin color, texture, response to dependency and elevation and the length of time for superficial wounds to heal should be noted. The femoral, popliteal and dorsalis pedis arteries are palpated and auscultated in the femoral triangle, popliteal fossa and dorsum of the foot respectively. If a deep vein thrombophlebitis is suspected, the response to passive dorsiflexion of the ankle should be noted (Homans' sign) and the region carefully palpated for heat and/or tenderness.

Soft tissue tests

The soft tissue overlying the lumbo-pelvic-hip region is palpated for signs of segmental facilitation which include:

1. the pilomotor reflex: 'goose flesh' in the dermatome of the facilitated segment
2. the sudomotor reflex: increased tendency for the skin to perspire in the dermatome of the facilitated segment
3. subcutaneous trophedema: 'peau d'orange' effect of segmentally facilitated subcutaneous tissue when it is rolled between the thumb and fingers
4. hypertonic musculature and reactive spasm: increased resting tone of the segmentally related spinal and peripheral musculature often associated with an increase in the myotatic reflex.

Local tenderness of the soft tissue to palpation is recorded and correlated' with the other objective findings.

Adjunctive tests

'X-rays make good policemen but poor counselors, in that while the straight radiography may exclude serious bone disease and significant mechanical defect, it does not often provide much guidance about how to treat the patient'.[48]

The primary reason, from the perspective of clinical manual therapy, for obtaining the results of adjunctive tests is to rule out serious pathology and to discover the presence of anatomical anomalies prior to the initiation of treatment.

The adjunctive tests available include the following:

1. radiography (X-rays)
2. discography
3. myelography
4. radiculography
5. epidurography
6. tomography
7. transverse axial tomography
8. computed transverse axial tomography
9. radiographic stereoplotting
10. interosseous spinal venography
11. cineradiography and fluoroscopy
12. thermography
13. nerve root infiltration
14. electrodiagnosis
15. intervertebral disc manometry
16. cystometry
17. radioactive isotope studies
18. ultrasonography
19. nuclear magnetic resonance.

With respect to the sacroiliac joint, Lawson et al[68] reported on the benefits of computed axial tomography (CT scanning techniques) as opposed to conventional radiography in the detection of mild erosions and narrowing of the joint. Because of the three-dimensional spatial orientation of the sacroiliac joint, CT scanning was superior in obtaining visualization of the joint space. Thus the diagnosis of inflammatory sacroiliitis, which is based on the identification of joint narrowing, sclerosis, ankylosis or erosion, was facilitated. Figures 7.42 to 7.45 illustrate the visualization of both the synovial and the ligamentous portions of the sacroiliac joint that is possible with this adjunctive test.

CT scanning techniques can reveal congenital and/or acquired anatomical changes at the lumbosacral junction (Fig. 7.46). The dimensions of the central spinal canal as well as the lateral recess are clearly visualized and often confirm or negate the clinical findings of physical trespass.

The lumbosacral junction is often the site of congenital anomalies which may or may not be significant to the clinical picture. Their presence, however, should be ascertained. The anomalies which are seen at this level include:[48]

1. asymmetry of the posterior zygapophysial joints

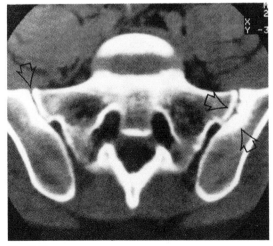

Fig. 7.42
(*Captions overleaf*)

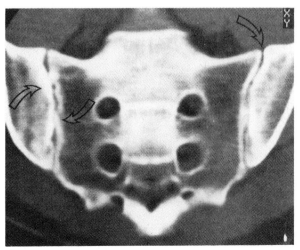

Fig. 7.43

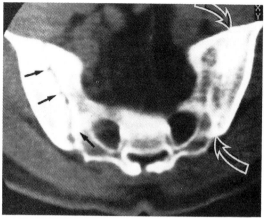

Fig. 7.44

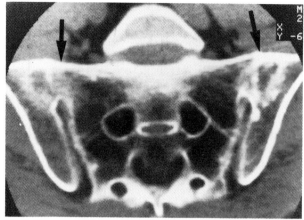

Fig. 7.45

Fig. 7.42   A computed tomography scan (transverse plane) of a patient with Reiter's disease. This technique clearly reveals the focal sclerosis (arrows), narrowing and erosion of the sacroiliac joint associated with this disease. The depth of the joint is clearly visualized.

Fig. 7.43   A computed tomography scan (vertical plane) of a patient with Reiter's disease illustrating narrowing, erosion and focal sclerosis (arrows) of the articular surfaces of the sacroiliac joints.

Fig. 7.44   A computed tomography scan of a patient with ankylosing spondylitis. Note the total ankylosis of the right sacroiliac joint (open arrows).

Fig. 7.45   A computed tomography scan of a patient with ankylosing spondylitis. Note the bilateral bony ankylosis of the sacroiliac joints.
   (Figures 7.42–7.45 are reproduced with permission from Lawson et al 1982 and the publishers Raven Press.)[68]

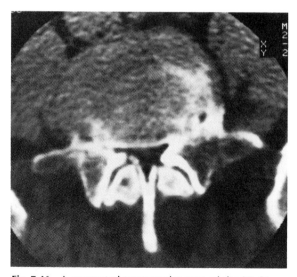

Fig. 7.46   A computed tomography scan of the L5–S1 segment illustrating central stenosis secondary to enlargement of the zygapophysial joints bilaterally. (Reproduced with permission from Kirkaldy-Willis 1983.)[65]

2. congenital absence of a pedicle
3. accessory laminae
4. osseous bridging of the transverse processes
5. dysplasia or absence of the spinous process of the L5 or S1 vertebrae (spina bifida)
6. dysplasia of the pars interarticularis
7. spina magna of the L5 vertebra
8. trapezoidal L5 vertebra, lumbarized S1 vertebra—partial or complete
9. sacralized L5 vertebra—partial or complete
10. anomalous adventitious joint between the transverse process of the L5 vertebra and the ala of the sacrum
11. asymmetric height of the ala of the sacrum with one side higher than the other creating a 'sacral tilt'
12. calcified iliolumbar ligament.

The findings noted on adjunctive testing of the lumbo-pelvic-hip complex must be correlated with the findings noted on clinical examination if their significance is to be understood. Rarely can treatment be directed by the results of these tests alone.

8

Lumbosacral junction: clinical syndromes

CLASSIFICATION

Lumbosacral disorders have been classified[78] as visceral, vascular, neurogenic, psychogenic, sociogenic and/or spondylogenic in origin. Briefly, disorders of the pelvic viscera can refer pain to the lumbosacral region and are easily confused with benign mechanical dysfunction. Insufficiency of the peripheral vascular system can secondarily give rise to backache and/or symptoms resembling sciatica. Neurogenic disorders include benign and/or malignant tumors of the central or peripheral nervous system. A central lesion at the lumbosacral junction can mimic a cauda equina compression lesion. Pure psychogenic or sociogenic backache is not often seen although stress can play a role in magnifying the perception of pain.

Spondylogenic disorders have been further classified[78] as:

1. Pathologic soft tissue and bony
   a. Scheuermann's disease—vertebral osteochondritis
   b. Infective—pyogenic vertebral osteomyelitis
   c. Systemic inflammatory—rheumatoid arthritis, ankylosing spondylitis
   d. Metabolic—osteoporosis, Paget's disease, tuberculosis, Calvé's disease, DISH (diffuse idiopathic skeletal hyperostosis)
2. Traumatic soft tissue and bony
   a. Fractures
   b. Contusions
   c. Spondylolisthesis/spondylolysis

3. Aging, adaptation, degeneration
   a. Arthrosis of the posterior zygapophysial joints
   b. Spondylosis of the intervertebral disc.

Systemic and/or inflammatory disorders affecting the lumbosacral region can be differentiated clinically from traumatic inflammation (i.e. sprain) by the lack of trauma in the history, the inconsistent response of the joint to both mechanical stress and to rest, as well as the lack of resolution with appropriate therapy over a short period of time. The experienced clinician will quickly recognize the pattern of response to therapy which deviates from the norm, and will question the biomechanical pathogenesis at this point. Subsequent investigation is then indicated.

Although scientific verification of the anatomical and physiological factors responsible for nociception are essential for specific diagnosis, prognosis and classifications such as those above, they rarely enhance our ability to treat the patient. For the clinical manual therapist, classifications which follow a biomechanical model based on mobility and stability have proven more useful and provide a consistent therapeutic approach. In keeping with this model, lumbosacral disorders can be classified into three groups, each of which describes the objective findings noted on mobility testing and suggests the appropriate restorative therapy. They include:
1. Hypomobility with or without pain
2. Hypermobility with or without pain
3. Normal mobility with pain.

This classification pertains to the presence or absence of osteokinematic function of the L5 vertebra relative to the sacrum and is directly dependent upon the composite arthrokinematic and myokinematic function of the L5–S1 articulation (see Ch. 5). This classification does not provide a specific anatomical nor physiological cause for the aberrant mobility noted; however, since mobilization and stabilization techniques used in manual therapy are specific to restoring movement patterns, the cause is not always required for formulating treatment plans. The aim of all evaluation procedures is to identify the system (i.e. articular v. myofascial) which is aberrantly altering the osteokinematic function of the L5 vertebra during functional movement. Subsequently, treatment can be directed to the articular and/or myofascial system. If the biomechanics of the lumbopelvic-hip region are restored in accordance with those presented in Chapter 5, symptomatic and objective improvement usually follows *if* the underlying etiology is biomechanical in nature.

HYPOMOBILITY WITH OR WITHOUT PAIN

The physiological and anatomical changes which accompany lumbosacral dysfunction in this category have been described and beautifully illustrated by Kirkaldy-Willis.[65,67] The essential objective finding for classification here is *decreased* osteokinematic motion of the L5 vertebra relative to the sacrum. The etiology of restriction may be either articular, myofascial or both and is commonly the result of an excessive rotational or compressive force which exceeded the kinematic range of the unit.[32,44,45,65,67]

The specific anatomical and physiological changes include:
1. synovitis of the posterior zygapophysial joints (Grade 1–2 sprain), strain of the iliolumbar ligament
2. minor circumferential tears of the outer layers of the annulus and the associated anterior and posterior longitudinal ligaments (Fig. 8.1)
3. minor joint subluxations
4. end-plate fractures (compression overload, rarely seen at the lumbosacral junction)[34,65]
5. hypertonic segmental posterior musculature.

Subjective findings

The mode of onset may be either insidious or sudden, depending upon the degree of trauma encountered. The presence or absence of pain is directly dependent upon mechanical and/or chemical irritation of the local nociceptors which in turn is a function of the stage

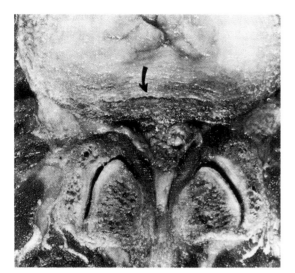

Fig. 8.1 A transverse circumferential tear in the annulus fibrosis (arrow). (Reproduced with permission from Kirkaldy-Willis 1983.)[65]

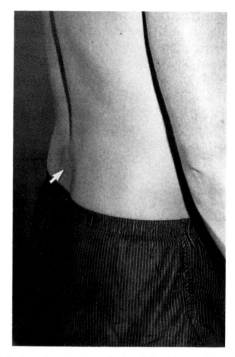

Fig. 8.2 Localized rotoscoliosis of the L5 vertebra (arrow) secondary to hypertonicity of the lumbar longissimus muscle.

of the pathology (substrate, fibroblastic, maturation). The pain may be unilateral or bilateral and is usually localized to the lumbosacral junction with occasional radiation to the buttock. Dysaesthesia is not often reported. The aggravating activities commonly include the extremes of range of motion of forward/backward bending, prolonged standing and lifting. Rest usually affords relief.

Objective findings

Mobility

In the first few days after injury (substrate phase), the patient with acute symptoms presents with marked restriction in all ranges of motion. Both forward and backward bending are limited as well as lateral bending to the left and right. The range of motion is bilaterally limited when the pathology is bilateral, and unilaterally limited when the pathology is unilateral. There may be a localized kyphosis and/or scoliosis evident at the lumbosacral junction (Fig. 8.2) secondary to the hypertonic lumbar longissimus muscle whose orientation (see Ch. 4) retracts the L5 vertebra.[15,16] The severity of the pain usually restricts a detailed mobility assessment at this

stage; however, with resolution over the next few days, mobility testing (see Ch. 7) confirms the restricted osteokinematic function of the L5–S1 segment.

During the fibroblastic stage, unilateral restrictions of flexion and/or extension may produce a multisegmental rotoscoliosis during forward and/or backward bending of the trunk, manifested both during the osteokinematic and positional testing of the lumbar spine. This is the first sign that an underlying restriction exists, since neither rotation nor sideflexion should occur coupled with flexion/extension during forward or backward bending of the trunk (in the presence of a level sacral base—see Ch. 5). The ipsilateral kinetic test may also be adversely effected by the hypomobile lesion (see Ch. 7).

In the initial stages of injury, arthrokinematic testing specific to the L5–S1 segment reveals a full range of articular motion. Palpation of the hypertonic segmental musculature confirms the myofascial etiology of the restriction. Treatment should be directed towards restoring the function of the myofascial system (active mobilization techniques).

If restrictive capsular adhesions develop, the arthrokinematic function will be reduced and confirmed on testing. Treatment should now be directed towards both the articular system (passive mobilization techniques) as well as the myofascial system (active mobilization techniques) for full restoration of function.

Stability

Lumbosacral disorders in this category do not exhibit a loss of arthrokinetic function. After the initial acute stage has subsided, the kinetic tests for compression, torsion and postero-anterior shear stability are normal.

Neurological tests

All tests for neurological conductivity and dural mobility relative to the lumbosacral junction are normal.

Classification of hypomobile dysfunction

The segmental restriction can be subclassified according to the position in which the L5 vertebra is held. A Flexed L5 vertebra exhibits a bilateral restriction of extension, whereas an Extended L5 vertebra exhibits a bilateral restriction of flexion. The unilateral lesions produce a segmental rotoscoliosis of the L5 vertebra as well as a compensatory multisegmental rotoscoliosis above the L5 vertebra. Consequently, a Flexed, Rotated/Sideflexed, Left (FRSL) L5 vertebra exhibits a restriction of extension and right rotation/sideflexion, whereas an Extended, Rotated/Sideflexed, Left (ERSL) L5 vertebra exhibits a restriction of flexion and right rotation/sideflexion. Note that this terminology does not identify the pathogenesis of the restriction.

Treatment of the hypomobile lumbosacral junction

Treatment of the lumbosacral junction forms part of the overall rehabilitation of the lumbo-pelvic-hip complex. The ultimate goal is to restore the optimal function of the entire unit both kinematically as well as kinetically, part of which requires the optimal function of the L5–S1 joint complex. The following section outlines the specific therapy indicated during each stage of repair (i.e. substrate, fibroblastic, maturation) when localized hypomobility of the L5–S1 joint complex is found.

The myofascial, postural and ergonomic components of therapy pertinent to the lumbo-pelvic-hip complex will be discussed in Chapter 11.

Substrate phase

During the first four to six days after injury, the goal of treatment is hemostasis of the wound. At home, the frequent application of ice together with rest is the treatment of choice.

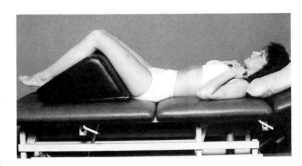

Fig. 8.3 The resting position of the lumbo-pelvic-hip complex.

The resting position of the lumbo-pelvic-hip complex (Fig. 8.3) is the supine position with the hips and knees semi-flexed and supported over a wedge. The surface should be firm, but not rigid.

At the clinic, electrotherapeutic analgesic modalities such as transcutaneous nerve stimulation and interferential current therapy can afford relief from pain; however, the patient should not attend at this stage if the physical stresses induced are greater than the relief gained.

Fibroblastic phase

With the resolution of active range of movement, the specific osteokinematic restriction becomes apparent. During this stage of repair, the goal of treatment is twofold, to restore the segmental articular mobility (kinematics) as well as the tensile strength of the unit (kinetics). Passive and active mobilization techniques are utilized to restore the articular kinematics, and combined with ultrasound and LASER for the enhancement of collagen production (tensile strength) at the wound site.[1,8,86,133] In addition, a specific home exercise program designed to maintain and increase articular mobility is given. Details of the treatment for two hypomobile lumbosacral dysfunctions in this stage of repair are outlined below.

Flexed rotated/sideflexed left (FRSL) L5–S1 joint complex

Specific traction—passive mobilization technique (Fig. 8.4). This is an extremely useful preliminary mobilization technique which can be graded according to the irritability of the joint. Initially, gentle grades are indicated, keeping well within the range of pain and reactive muscle spasm. The large afferent fiber input from the Type I and II mechanoreceptors located in the articular capsule inhibits

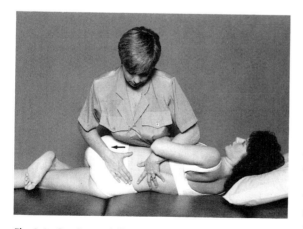

Fig. 8.4 Passive mobilization—specific traction of the lumbosacral junction. The arrow indicates the direction of force applied to the patient's pelvic girdle.

the centripetal transmission of the small fiber input (nociception) at the spinal cord, thus reducing the perception of pain via the spinal gating mechanism (see Ch. 4).

The stimulation of the Type I and II mechanoreceptors also reduces the gamma efferent discharge to the intrafusal muscle fiber of the segmentally related muscle, thus reducing hypertonicity. If the myofascia is primarily responsible for the restriction of osteokinematic function, this technique should certainly be included in the early treatment plan.

With the patient sidelying, hips and knees slightly flexed, the interspinous space between the L4 and the L5 vertebra is palpated with the caudal hand. The thoracolumbar spine is rotated by pulling the patient's lower arm forward until full rotation of the L4–L5 joint complex is achieved. The cranial hand now palpates the interspinous space between the L5 vertebra and the sacrum while the caudal hand flexes the patient's uppermost hip and knee. Simultaneously, the patient should extend the lower leg to the end of the table. The foot of the upper leg is allowed to rest against the popliteal fossa of the lower leg. The therapist's lower lateral thorax contacts the patient's uppermost innominate bone.

Specific traction is applied to the lumbosacral junction via a straight caudal force from the therapist's lower lateral thorax against the patient's pelvic girdle. The therapist's cranial arm stabilizes the patient's upper thorax. The degree of force applied is dictated by the joint/myofascial reaction.

Rotation/sideflexion—passive and active mobilization techniques. The rotation/sideflexion component of the osteokinematic restriction is usually myofascial in origin at this stage of repair since restrictive capsular adhesions have not had time to form. Grades 2 and 3[48] rotation/sideflexion passive mobilization techniques are utilized for their neurophysiological effect on the segmental myofascia, that is the reduction in hypertonicity and subsequently the return of osteokinematic function. The technique yields the best result when it is used in combination with the active mobilization technique (vide infra).

Localization. With the patient in left side-lying, hips and knees slightly flexed, the interspinous space between the L4 and the L5 vertebra is palpated with the caudal hand. The thoracolumbar spine is rotated by pulling the patient's lower arm forward until full rotation of the L4–L5 joint complex is achieved. The cranial hand now palpates the interspinous space between the L5 vertebra and the sacrum while the caudal hand flexes the patient's uppermost hip and knee. Simultaneously, the patient should extend the lower leg to the end of the table. The foot of the upper leg is allowed to rest against the popliteal fossa of the lower leg. The therapist's cranial arm supports the patient's thorax while the caudal arm supports the pelvic girdle.

Passive mobilization (Fig. 8.5). From the above described position, the L5–S1 joint complex is passively mobilized into extension and right rotation/sideflexion about the appropriate *oblique* axis (see Ch. 5) through either the thorax or the pelvic girdle. The technique is graded in accordance with the joint/myofascial reaction.

Active mobilization (Fig. 8.6). The L5–S1 joint complex is initially mobilized passively into extension and right rotation/sideflexion about the appropriate oblique axis, through either the thorax or the pelvic girdle, to the limit of the physiological range of motion. In this position, the patient is instructed to resist further motion while the therapist applies a gentle rotation force to the pelvic girdle or the

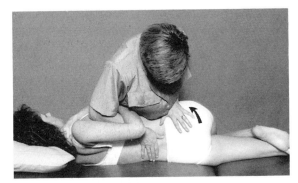

Fig. 8.6 Active mobilization for extension and right rotation/sideflexion of the lumbosacral junction. The arrow indicates the direction of resistance applied by the therapist.

thorax. The isometric contraction is held for up to five seconds followed by a period of complete relaxation. The joint is then passively taken to the new physiological range of extension and right rotation/side flexion. The technique is repeated three times followed by re-evaluation of osteokinematic function.

Home exercise program. A home exercise program designed to restore segmental osteokinematic function at the lumbosacral junction is paramount to successful rehabilitation. Since wound repair occurs throughout 24 h, the orientation of the newly formed collagen fibers should be directed as often as possible (see Ch. 6).

In the early fibroblastic stage of repair, gentle range of motion exercises well within the painfree range are indicated. The hypo-

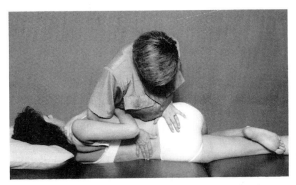

Fig. 8.5 Passive mobilization for extension and right rotation/sideflexion of the lumbosacral junction.

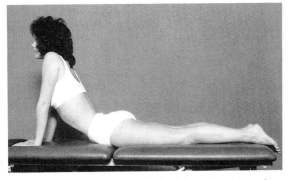

Fig. 8.7 Passive press-ups, the initial exercise given for mobilization of the FRSL lesion, should be repeated six times, six times per day.

mobile lumbosacral junction which is held in
the flexed, left rotated/sideflexed (FRSL)
position requires an exercise program aimed
at restoring extension and right
rotation/sideflexion. Passive press-up (Fig. 8.7)
from the prone position repeated six times,
six times per day are the initial exercises
given. Subsequently, unilateral left leg raises
from the prone position (Fig. 8.8) producing
intra-pelvic torsion and right lumbosacral rotation (see Ch. 5), can be added.

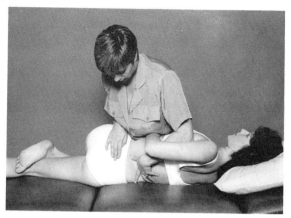

Fig. 8.9 Passive mobilization for flexion and left
rotation/sideflexion of the lumbosacral junction.

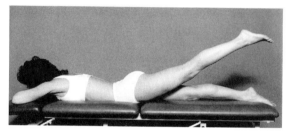

Fig. 8.8 Unilateral left leg raises for mobilization of the
FRSL lesion.

Extended rotated/sideflexed right (ERSR) L5–S1 joint complex

*Specific traction—passive mobilization tech-
nique (Fig. 8.4).* As with the FRSL lesion,
specific traction is an extremely useful preliminary mobilization technique which can be
graded according to the irritability of the joint.
The details and the intent of this technique
are identical to those described above.

*Rotation/sideflexion—passive and active
mobilization techniques.* See the FRSL lesion
for details on the intent of these techniques
during the fibroblastic stage of repair.

Localization. With the patient in right sidelying, hips and knees slightly flexed, the interspinous space between the L4 and the L5
vertebra is palpated with the caudal hand. The
thoracolumbar spine is rotated by pulling the
patient's lower arm until full rotation of the
L4–L5 joint complex is achieved. The cranial
hand now palpates the interspinous space
between the L5 vertebra and the sacrum while
the caudal hand flexes the patient's uppermost hip and knee. Simultaneously, the

patient should extend the lower leg to the
end of the table. The foot of the upper leg is
allowed to rest against the popliteal fossa of
the lower leg. The therapist cranial arm
supports the patient's thorax while the caudal
arm supports the pelvic girdle.

Passive mobilization (Fig. 8.9). From the
above described position, the L5–S1 joint
complex is passively mobilized into flexion
and left rotation/sideflexion about the appropriate *oblique* axis (see Ch. 5) through either
the thorax or the pelvic girdle. The technique is graded in accordance with the joint/
myofascial reaction.

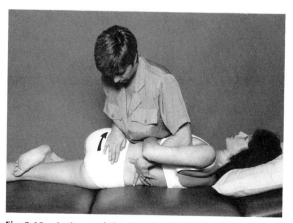

Fig. 8.10 Active mobilization for flexion and left
rotation/sideflexion of the lumbosacral junction. The
arrow indicates the direction of resistance applied by
the therapist.

Active mobilization (Fig. 8.10). The L5–S1 joint complex is initially mobilized passively into flexion and left rotation/sideflexion about the appropriate oblique axis, through either the thorax or the pelvic girdle, to the limit of the physiological range of motion. In this position, the patient is instructed to resist further motion while the therapist applies a gentle rotation force to the pelvic girdle or the thorax. The isometric contraction is held for up to five seconds followed by a period of complete relaxation. The joint is then passively taken to the new physiological range of flexion and left rotation/sideflexion. The technique is repeated three times followed by re-evaluation of osteokinematic function.

Home exercise program. A home exercise program designed to restore segmental osteokinematic function at the lumbosacral junction is paramount to successful rehabilitation. Since wound repair occurs throughout 24 h, the orientation of the newly formed collagen fibers should be directed as often as possible (see Ch. 6).

In the early fibroblastic stage of repair, gentle range of motion exercises well within the painfree range, are indicated. The hypomobile lumbosacral junction which is held in the extended, right rotated/sideflexed (ERSR) position requires an exercise program aimed at restoring flexion and left rotation/sideflexion. Passive curl-ups (Fig. 8.11) from the supine position repeated six times, six times

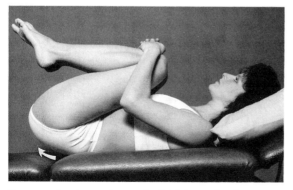

Fig. 8.11 Passive curl-ups, the initial exercise for mobilization of the ERSR lesion, should be repeated six times, six times per day.

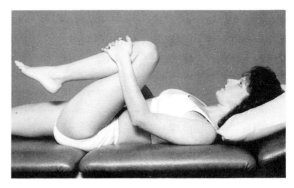

Fig. 8.12 Unilateral flexion of the left hip in the supine position for mobilization of the ERSR lesion.

per day are the initial exercises given. Subsequently, unilateral flexion of the left hip (Fig. 8.12) in the supine position producing intrapelvic torsion and left lumbosacral rotation (see Ch. 5), can be added.

Maturation phase

If restrictive capsular adhesions have developed during the fibroblastic stage of repair, stronger passive mobilization techniques will be required to restore the optimal kinematic function of the lumbosacral junction. In addition, a vigorous home exercise program designed to reorganize the collagen fibers within the adhesion will be necessary.

The active and passive mobilization techniques utilized at this stage of repair are identical to those previously described except that the joint is taken strongly and specifically to the limit of the physiological range of motion (Grade 4). Grade 5 (high velocity, low amplitude thrust) techniques are indicated when the joint irritability is low and the end feel of motion is very hard. The localization and positioning for the Grade 5 technique is identical to that previously described. The direction of the thrust is critical to the success of the technique and must be about the appropriate oblique axis of rotation. Unfortunately, it is impossible to learn from a book the feel of the indications and the direction of 'thrust' that is required in this technique.

The specific exercises given in the maturation stage of repair are identical to those described above with the exception that they need not be contained within the painfree range of motion; however, the quality of the pain induced as well as its duration should be minimal. Exercises for global lumbo-pelvic-hip function (see Ch. 11) should also be included.

Case history

A 27-year-old warehouse worker presented at the clinic two days after the onset of low back pain following a heavy day of repetitive lifting and twisting. During one such lift, he noted an acute twinge of pain in his low back which forced him to remain in a kyphotic position for several minutes. Eventually he was able to straighten up and immediately reported for first aid. Subsequent to seeing his family physician, he was referred to physiotherapy for evaluation and treatment.

This was the first episode of low back pain which had forced his absence from work. He had experienced low back pain in the past from which he had been able to recover spontaneously with rest. The pain was located at the lumbosacral junction with bilateral radiation into both buttocks. Dysaesthesia was not reported. The aggravating factors included all extremes of motion, in particular, forward bending.

Initially, objective examination was limited by the severity of the pain evoked on movement testing. Osteokinematically, all motions of the lumbo-pelvic-hip complex were restricted. Over the next few days, as the acute inflammatory stage (substrate phase) subsided, the habitual movement tests revealed an asymmetry of motion of the L5 vertebra relative to the sacrum on forward bending such that the right transverse process travelled further superiorly than the left. Subsequent regional osseous/articular mobility tests exposed a segmental restriction of flexion and right rotation of the L5–S1 joint complex. The arthrokinetic and neurological tests were normal. The segmental musculature was hypertonic to palpation and reactive to stretch, suggesting a myofascial etiology. This lesion can be classified as an ERSL—the joint is held in a position of extension and rotation/sideflexion to the left and limited in flexion and rotation/sideflexion to the right.

The patient was advised to rest in the supine position with a wedge or support beneath the semi-flexed knees and to apply ice to the lumbar spine frequently. On the sixth day after injury gentle passive and active mobilization was begun. The techniques chosen included specific traction, passive flexion and right rotation/sideflexion combined with an active mobilization in the same direction. Interferential current therapy was given as an electrotherapeutic analgesic and the patient was sent home with gentle flexion exercises (curl-ups) to be kept well within the painfree range.

The patient was seen three times weekly over the next three weeks during which the lumbosacral junction was progressively mobilized until optimal osteokinematic function had returned. At least six months of healing time is required before the tensile strength of the damaged tissue is restored; therefore, careful review of proper ergonomics (see Ch. 11) was a crucial part of this patient's rehabilitation.

HYPERMOBILITY WITH OR WITHOUT PAIN

Repeated trauma to the lumbosacral junction can result in progressive anatomical and

Table 8.1 The degenerative process (from Kirkaldy-Willis 1983)[65]

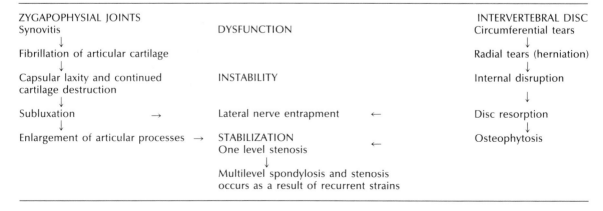

ZYGAPOPHYSIAL JOINTS		INTERVERTEBRAL DISC
Synovitis	DYSFUNCTION	Circumferential tears
↓		↓
Fibrillation of articular cartilage		Radial tears (herniation)
↓		↓
Capsular laxity and continued cartilage destruction	INSTABILITY	Internal disruption
↓		↓
Subluxation →	Lateral nerve entrapment ←	Disc resorption
↓		↓
Enlargement of articular processes →	STABILIZATION One level stenosis	← Osteophytosis
	↓	
	Multilevel spondylosis and stenosis occurs as a result of recurrent strains	

physiological changes which have been categorized by Kirkaldy-Willis[65,67] as the second stage of degeneration—instability (Table 8.1). The essential objective finding for classification here is the presence of *increased* osteokinematic motion of the L5 vertebra relative to the sacrum.

Following extreme or repeated rotational and/or posteroanterior shear trauma, the following anatomical and physiological changes can occur:

1. fibrillation and subsequent loss of the articular cartilage of the zygapophysial joint(s) (Figs 8.13, 8.14)
2. laxity of the articular capsule(s) and attenuation of the iliolumbar ligament
3. fracture of the articular process with resultant strain deformation of the neural arch
4. coalescence of the circumferential annular tears into a radial fissure (Fig. 8.15) with/without subsequent herniation of the nucleus pulposus, ultimately progressing to marked internal disruption of the disc, loss of disc height, circumferential bulging and resorption
5. sclerosis of the adjacent vertebral bodies (Fig. 8.16).

At the lumbosacral junction, these anatomical changes allow the superior articular process of the sacrum to sublux upwards and

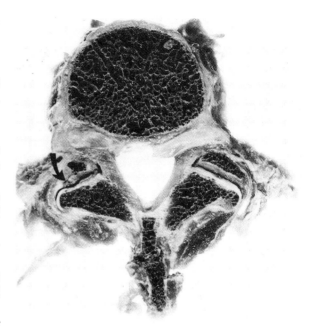

Fig. 8.14 Macroscopic transverse section of the L5–S1 segment. Note the marked degeneration of the left zygapophysial joint (arrow).

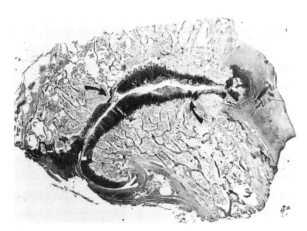

Fig. 8.13 Histological section of the zygapophysial joint. Note the thinning and fibrillation of the articular cartilage (arrows).

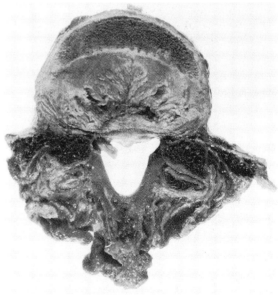

Fig. 8.15 Macroscopic transverse section of the L4–L5 segment. Note the coalescence of several radial fissures and the early stages of internal disruption. (Figs 8.13, 8.14 and 8.15 reproduced with permission from Kirkaldy-Willis 1983.)[65]

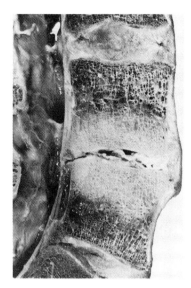

Fig. 8.16 Macroscopic sagittal section of the lumbar spine. Note the sclerosis of the vertebral bodies above and below the central intervertebral disc which is markedly resorbed. (Reproduced with permission from Kirkaldy-Willis et al 1978.)[67]

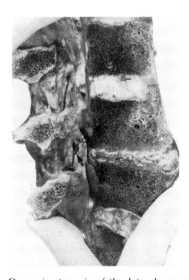

Fig. 8.17 Dynamic stenosis of the lateral recess of the lumbosacral junction associated with instability. In this specimen the spinous process of the L5 vertebra has been rotated towards the observer. The zygapophysial joint has opened (arrow), the superior articular process has approximated the posterior aspect of the intervertebral disc subsequently narrowing the lateral recess. (Reproduced with permission from Reilly J, et al 1978.)[100]

forwards during axial rotation of the trunk (Fig. 8.17). This motion consequently narrows the lateral recess of the L5–S1 joint complex, potentially impeding the vascular and neurological function of the structures within the intervertebral foramen.[115] This is referred to as dynamic instability or dynamic stenosis.[65]

Subjective findings

Clinically, the patient with a hypermobile lumbosacral junction presents with a long history of intermittent low back pain with repeat episodes of exacerbation and resolution. The presence or absence of pain is dependent upon mechanical and/or chemical irritation of the local nociceptors, as well as the individual's overall level of mobility. The pain may be unilateral or bilateral and can be referred as far as the distal extent of the L5 or S1 dermatome. Dysaesthesia is common, given the potential for neurovascular impedance at the intervertebral foramen. The aggravating activities depend upon which anatomical structure is currently responsible for nociceptive transmission. Disorders of the neural arch frequently resemble the hypomobile lesion subjectively in that extreme ranges of motion, lifting and prolonged standing can be aggravating activities. When the intervertebral disc is responsible for pain production, compressive activities such as prolonged sitting and flexion are intolerable. Rest usually affords relief.

Objective findings

Mobility

Objectively, the hypermobile patient may adopt altered lumbo-pelvic-hip movement patterns to compensate for the loss of kinetic stability at the lumbosacral junction. Typically, they forward bend by walking their hands down their thighs and back up to return to erect standing (Fig. 8.18). Alternately, they may forward and backward bend by utilizing the osteokinematic function of the pelvic girdle on the hip joints without involving the

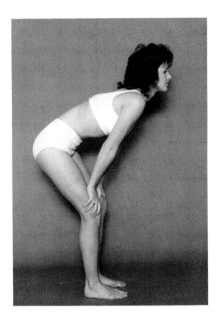

Fig. 8.18 Typical pattern of forward bending of the trunk when arthrokinetic stability is lost at the lumbosacral junction.

spinal segments at all. Often, a deep skin crease is noted at the unstable level during backward bending of the trunk (Fig. 8.19). The normal lumbo-pelvic-hip rhythm during functional movement may even be reversed (see Ch. 5).

Specific mobility testing of the lumbosacral junction reveals increased mobility of flexion/extension and/or sideflexion/rotation.

The presence or absence of pain on these tests is dependent upon the level of irritability of the joint at the time of evaluation. Commonly, a patient with acute low back pain will initially present with a hypomobile segment due to the reactive muscle spasm. With resolution, the underlying hypermobile joint is revealed.

Stability

The kinetic tests for posteroanterior shear and torsion stability are always positive for pain and excess range of motion in the pathological, hypermobile, lumbosacral segment.

Neurological tests

Impedance of neurological function (motor, sensory, reflex) and dural mobility is common in patients with hypermobility (instability). Laterally, dynamic instability interferes with the dimensions of the lateral recess, poten-

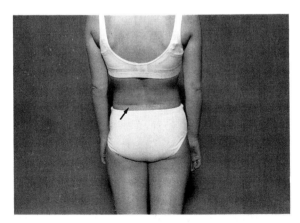

Fig. 8.19 When segmental hypermobility of anteroposterior translation is present, backward bending of the trunk will produce a localized deep skin crease (arrow).

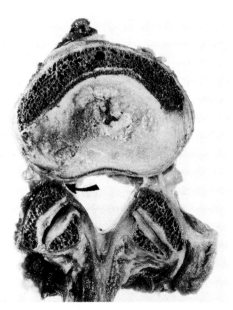

Fig. 8.20 Macroscopic transverse section of the L4–L5 segment demonstrating the effect of instability on the dimensions of the lateral recess. Note the approximation of the superior articular process towards the intervertebral disc on the left during axial rotation and the subsequent obliteration of the left lateral recess (arrow). (Reproduced with permission from Kirkaldy-Willis 1983.)[65]

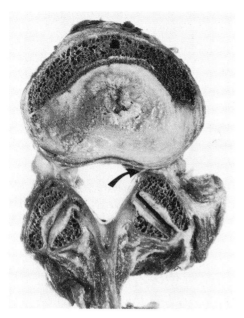

Fig. 8.21 The same specimen as in Figure 8.20 axially rotated in the opposite direction. Note the approximation of the superior articular process towards the intervertebral disc on the right (compare with Figure 8.20) and the subsequent obliteration of the right lateral recess (arrow). (Reproduced with permission from Kirkaldy-Willis 1983.)[65]

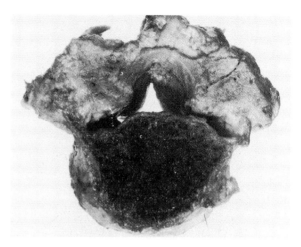

Fig. 8.22 Macroscopic transverse section of the L5–S1 segment illustrating fixed central and lateral stenosis. The central and lateral canals are markedly narrowed by osteophytosis. (Reproduced with permission from Kirkaldy-Willis 1983.)[65]

tially impeding the neurovascular bundle (Figs 8.20, 8.21). At the lumbosacral junction, the L5 nerve root would be effected. Centrally, the nucleus pulposus or the annulus can herniate thus reducing the dimensions of the spinal canal and consequently interfere with the S1 nerve root. In both instances, the straight leg raise test for dural mobility would be adversely effected.

The spectrum of neurological impedance is variable, depending upon the degree of pathology. The patient may present with minimal motor weakness or sensory dysaesthesia in the early stages, and later with a complete motor nerve block and sensory anaesthesia. Careful objective evaluation is mandatory to detect the early neurological decompensation.

End results

With time, the posterior zygapophysial joints enlarge to develop osteophytes, the interver-

tebral disc becomes fibrotic and traction spurs may develop on the anterior and/or posterior aspect of the vertebral body, occasionally leading to spontaneous fusion (Figs 8.22, 8.23). These changes occur during the third stage of the degenerative process, stabilization, and the patient is often painfree (as well as hypomobile).[65] The risk at this stage is the development of fixed central and/or lateral stenosis due to osseous trespass on the spinal canal and/or lateral recess with attendant peripheral symptoms of neurogenic vascular claudication.[115]

Treatment of the hypermobile lumbosacral junction

Treatment of the hypermobile lumbosacral junction forms part of the overall rehabilitation of the lumbo-pelvic-hip complex. The ultimate goal is to restore the optimal function of the entire unit both kinematically as well as kinetically, which requires the optimal function of the L5–S1 joint complex. The following section outlines the therapy indicated during the substrate and the fibroblastic stage of repair when localized hypermobility of the L5–S1 joint complex is found.

The myofascial, postural and ergonomic

Fibroblastic phase

With the resolution of active range of movement, the hypermobile lumbosacral junction becomes apparent. During this stage of repair, treatment is dependent upon which tissues have lost their kinetic ability and whether or not neurological impedance has occurred.

If used at all, specific mobilization techniques must be carefully applied and kept well within the physiological range of motion since it is stability, not mobility, that is required. Some clinicians use mobilization techniques as analgesic tools (e.g. for the neurophysiological effects of large afferent fiber stimulation on nociception); however, the electrotherapeutic modalities available today serve the same purpose. Ultrasound should be given at this stage for its influence on collagen production. Clinically, it appears that LASER can be an effective treatment at this time.

If impedance of the motor and/or sensory nerve roots is present, intermittent mechanical traction is indicated. The poundage required is that which is necessary to separate the joint, and the usual treatment time is 15 minutes with hold and rest periods of 10 seconds each. The neurological tests as well as the dural mobility tests are used as the objective guides to the success of the treatment and should be monitored before and after each treatment session.

The tests for stability to compression, torsion and shear are repeated frequently to assess the patient's progress. However, if the degree of trauma and subsequent kinetic decompensation has been significant, progress will be slow since the restoration of kinetic function requires 6 to 18 months of healing time (see Ch. 6). During this time, or if the loss of kinetic strength is permanent (Kirkaldy-Willis[65,67] stage 2—instability phase—of the degenerative process), postural and ergonomic retraining becomes the crux of therapy (see Ch. 11).

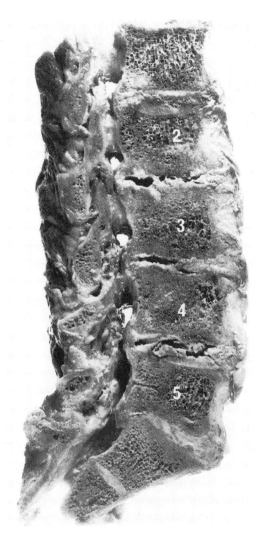

Fig. 8.23 Macroscopic sagittal section of the lumbar spine illustrating multilevel spinal stenosis. (Reproduced with permission from Kirkaldy-Willis 1983.)[65]

components of therapy are crucial to the rehabilitation of the hypermobile lumbosacral junction and will be discussed in Chapter 11.

Substrate phase

During the first four to six days after injury, the goal of treatment is hemostasis of the wound. At home, the frequent application of ice together with rest is the treatment of choice.

Case history

A 38-year-old carpenter presented at the clinic three weeks after the recurrence of low back pain. He had experienced multiple episodes of lumbosacral pain in the past, some of which had required time off work and medical attention. This episode developed following a 12-hour drive which had necessitated prolonged periods of sitting in a kyphotic position. Over the next three weeks, the local lumbosacral pain had spread distally into the right buttock, posterior thigh and leg to the mid-calf. Dysaesthesia was not reported. The major aggravating factors included forward bending and sitting in kyphosis. Walking and rest both afforded some relief.

Objectively, the habitual movement pattern of the lumbo-pelvic-hip complex was reversed such that during forward bending of the trunk the lumbar spine remained extended while the pelvic girdle flexed forward on the femoral heads. Although no support was required during forward bending, the patient returned to erect standing by supporting the weight of his trunk with his hands on his thighs.

Arthrokinetically, both the local and the referred pain was easily reproduced with passive compression as well as passive torsion to the right. The dural mobility of the L4 to S1 nerve roots was restricted to 45° by pain and reactive hamstring muscle spasm. The clinical neurological tests were normal for both motor and sensory conductivity.

As resolution occurred and specific mobility testing was possible, an underlying hypermobile L5–S1 joint complex was revealed. The hypermobility was apparent in flexion, right rotation and anterior translation. The compression strength gradually returned. This is a common pattern of early presentation of the hypermobile patient, who initially presents without 'hard' neurological signs but who is definitely at risk for future decompensation given the loss of arthrokinetic stability.

Treatment in the early stages included electrotherapeutic analgesic modalities for pain reduction and intermittent mechanical traction aimed at restoring the dural mobility. Postural and ergonomic retraining was the focus of therapy.

NORMAL MOBILITY WITH PAIN

Rotation sprains are most commonly seen at the L4–L5 segment since the iliolumbar ligament protects the lumbosacral junction against rotational trauma.[16,73] However, this ligament ties the L5 vertebra directly to the adjacent innominate bone which increases the risk of secondary breakdown as a consequence of altered function of this bone.

Clinically, the patient presents with localized pain at the lumbosacral junction which is easily exacerbated by palpation. However, careful objective evaluation of mobility reveals normal kinematic and kinetic function. The only biomechanical cause for this dysfunction is overuse of the articular and myofascial tissues in compensation for altered function elsewhere. Although local treatment may be required for pain reduction, correction of the global lumbo-pelvic-hip biomechanics is necessary for the prevention of recurrence. Alternately, the patient may have a disorder which is not biomechanical in nature, a possibility of which the clinician must always be aware.

9

The pelvic girdle: clinical syndromes

CLASSIFICATION

At the turn of this century, practitioners believed that the sacroiliac joint was the major source of sciatica admitting that, as well as sciatica, 'lumbago [and] backache . . . were frequently caused by an abnormal amount of motion in the pelvic joints, especially the sacroiliac synchondrosis'.[83] Aside from trauma, the influence of poor posture as well as lumbo-pelvic adaptation to extrinsic factors were recognized as being integral to the etiology of decompensation.

> The etiology of the pelvic joint conditions is not always clear, but there are many features of definite importance. At times the lesion apparently represents simply an excess of a normal physiological process. At other times trauma is a definite factor, 'sitting down hard', or the 'giving way' under severe strains, such as lifting, being the two most common forms of injury. Attitudes or postures are also of importance in causing or predisposing to joint weakness or displacement.[42]

The causes of mechanical pelvic girdle dysfunction remain the same today.

Aside from mechanical trauma, there are a number of conditions which can affect the pelvic girdle secondary to systemic disease. The majority of these are listed in Table 9.1. The reader is referred to the excellent article by Bellamy, Park and Rooney[10] for a concise description of the conditions tabulated.

The classifications for mechanical pelvic girdle dysfunction are multiple and usually describe restricted osteokinematic function of

Table 9.1 Conditions affecting the sacroiliac joint[10]

Inflammatory disorders
  Ankylosing spondylitis
  Reiter's syndrome
  Inflammatory bowel disease
  Psoriatic spondylitis
  Rheumatoid arthritis
  Juvenile rheumatoid arthritis
  Pustulotic arthroosteitis
  Familial Mediterranean fever
  Behçet's syndrome
  Relapsing polychondritis
  Whipple's disease
Joint infection
  Pyogenic
  Brucellosis
  Tuberculosis
Metabolic disorders
  Gout
  Calcium pyrosphosphate deposition disease
  Hyperparathyroidism
Miscellaneous
  Osteitis condensans ilii
  Paget's disease
  Acroosteolysis in polyvinyl chloride workers
  Alkaptonuria
  Gaucher's disease
  Tuberous sclerosis

either the sacrum or the innominate bone. Subsequently, labels such as 'posterior innominate', 'anterior sacrum', 'forward sacral torsion' and 'upslips' have emerged with little regard to universal nomenclature. The difficulty with this method of classification arises when interdisciplinary communication is attempted.

For the clinical manual therapist, classifications which follow a biomechanical model based on mobility and stability have proven more useful in facilitating a consistent approach to treatment and can be easily communicated to other health disciplines. In keeping with this model, pelvic girdle disorders can be classified into three groups, each of which describes the objective findings noted on mobility testing and suggests the appropriate restorative therapy. They include:
1. Hypomobility with or without pain
2. Hypermobility with or without pain
3. Normal mobility with pain.

This classification pertains to the presence or absence of osteokinematic function of the sacrum/innominate bones and is directly dependent upon the composite arthrokinematic and myokinematic function of the pelvic girdle (see Ch. 5). This classification does not provide a specific anatomical nor physiological cause for the aberrant mobility noted; however, since mobilization and stabilization techniques used in manual therapy are specific to restoring movement patterns, the cause is not always required for formulating treatment plans. The aim of all evaluation procedures is to identify the system (i.e. articular v. myofascial) which is aberrantly altering the osteokinematic function of the sacrum/innominate bones during functional movement. Subsequently, treatment can be directed towards the articular and/or the myofascial system. When the underlying etiology is biomechanical in nature, if the biomechanics of the lumbo-pelvic-hip region are restored to accord with those presented in Chapter 5, symptomatic and objective improvement usually follows.

HYPOMOBILITY WITH OR WITHOUT PAIN

Several authors of note have reported on their clinical findings of hypomobile pelvic girdle disorders.[3,9,36,37,38,63,88,89] The essential objective finding for classification here is *decreased* osteokinematic motion of either the sacrum or the innominate bone.

Subjective findings

The mode of onset may be either insidious or sudden depending upon the degree of trauma encountered. Typically, a fall on the buttocks or other direct injury can be found in the patient's history. The irritability of the sacroiliac joint during movement testing is dictated by the stage of pathology, the nature of the injury and the degree of inflammation present at the time of examination. The pain is usually localized to the sacroiliac joint and/or pubic symphysis; however, it may radiate through the pelvis to the anterior aspect of the ipsilateral groin and/or down the posterolateral buttock and thigh to the knee. Dysaesthesia is not often reported. The aggravating activities commonly include:

1. walking
2. stair climbing/descent
3. rolling over in bed
4. getting in/out of chair/car
5. one legged stance.

These patients commonly report an inability to find comfort in any one position or activity for a prolonged period of time and require frequent alterations in posture for relief. Although rest usually affords relief, asymmetric sleeping postures are often the ones of comfort.

Objective findings

Mobility

The pelvic girdle as a unit is capable of motion in all three body planes. During forward bending of the trunk in the sagittal plane, the innominate bones rotate about an anteroposterior oblique axis such that the iliac crests and the PSISs approximate while the ischial tuberosities and the ASISs separate (see Fig. 5.13). However, relative to one another there is no *intra-pelvic* torsion of the innominate bones. Sacral flexion between the innominate bones occurs purely (i.e. without torsion) during forward bending of the trunk. In the presence of unilateral hypomobility (with or without pain), forward bending of the trunk while standing produces intra-pelvic torsion of the innominate bones and/or sacrum. The presence of this finding should direct the examiner to a further detailed evaluation of the osteokinematic, arthrokinematic and myokinematic function of the pelvic girdle.

During backward bending of the trunk in the sagittal plane, the innominate bones simultaneously rotate about an anteroposterior oblique axis such that the iliac crests and the PSISs separate while the ischial tuberosities and the ASISs approximate (see Fig. 5.15). However, relative to one another there is no *intra-pelvic* torsion of the innominate bones. Sacral extension between the innominate bones occurs purely (i.e. without torsion) during backward bending of the trunk. Again, in the presence of unilateral hypomobility (with or without pain), backward bending of the trunk produces intra-pelvic torsion of the innominate bones and/or sacrum and should direct the examiner to a further detailed evaluation of the kinematic function of the pelvic girdle.

Translation of the pelvic girdle in the coronal plane during lateral bending of the trunk normally produces *intra-pelvic* torsion of the innominate bones and the sacrum (see Fig. 5.17). When unilateral hypomobility exists, fluent lateral bending of the body is inhibited and the 'hip shift' (ability to translate the pelvic girdle in the coronal plane without deviation—see Fig. 5.16) is subsequently lost or altered. Consequently, the pelvic girdle is not displaced lateral to the pedal base and increased muscular effort both from the trunk and the lower extremities is required to maintain balance.

The hypomobile sacroiliac joint can also be detected via the striding tests (ipsilateral kinetic test in standing and lying prone). The restriction becomes apparent as a reduction or total absence of relative motion between the innominate bone and the sacrum during one or both of the tests.

Stability

Pelvic girdle disorders in this category do not exhibit a loss of arthrokinetic function.

Muscle function—myokinematics

Apart from specific articular lesions, alterations in muscle function also play a role in the pathogenesis of hypomobile lumbo-pelvic-hip disorders. Janda has observed[56,57,58] that certain muscle groups respond to nociceptive stimulus by increasing tightness (postural muscles) while others respond by progressive weakness (phasic muscles).

Whatever the physiological basis for these changes of muscle function, the clinical fact remains that a developed muscle imbalance should be treated and that muscles in which we find a predominantly static or postural function and which show a tendency to get tight are activated in various movement patterns relatively more than muscles with a predominantly dynamic, phasic function, which show a tendency to get weak.[57]

Grieve notes that the more established the altered muscle pattern, the more disturbed the functional movement pattern becomes. 'The genesis of painful, degenerative joint conditions may frequently lie in more regional, and major, chronic imbalance of functional movement patterns, which place sustained and abnormal stress on joints'.[48]

Thus it is imperative to remember that although the assessment and treatment of the articular components of the lumbo-pelvic-hip region is emphasized, the motor system functions as a whole and the abnormal movement patterns may persist long after the articular function has been restored. Rehabilitation is incomplete until this component is addressed.

Relative to the pelvic girdle, the postural muscles which tend to tighten include the:
1. erector spinae/quadratus lumborum
2. hamstrings
3. rectus femoris
4. iliopsoas
5. tensor fascia lata
6. adductors
7. piriformis.

The phasic muscles which tend to weaken include the:
1. abdominals
2. gluteus maximus, medius, minimus
3. vastus medialis, lateralis, intermedius.

Clinically, myofascial imbalances exhibit a restriction or deviation of habitual movement *in the presence of normal articular mobility.*

Neurological tests

Impedance of neurological function and/or dural mobility can occur and is dependent upon the degree of decompensation of the lumbosacral junction (see Ch. 8—hypermobile disorders) as a consequence of the pelvic girdle dysfunction.

Classification of hypomobile dysfunction

Unilateral restriction of the innominate bone and/or sacrum can be subclassified according to the position in which the restricted bone is held. The following restrictions are commonly seen in clinical practice.

Flexed/laterally rotated innominate bone (posteriorly rotated/outflared)

Subjective findings. The mode of onset is usually traumatic. Commonly, the patient reports that one leg slipped out from under them, or that they stepped unexpectedly off a curb. An overzealous kick against a missed target is another frequent etiology. Pregnancy appears to predispose the pelvis to this disorder although major trauma does not usually play a role.

The pain is usually localized to the sacroiliac joint and can vary from acute, sharp and stabbing to a deep, dull ache, depending upon the stage of pathology. If the history is long, the painful side may not be the hypomobile one and careful objective examination is required to identify the side of the restriction. The aggravating activities include unilateral weight-bearing (the limb may be constantly postured in flexion), walking, lying supine with the extremity straight, and any activity requiring extension of the pelvic girdle.

Objective findings. The patient's altered gait pattern is often the first sign observed. The stride length is characteristically shortened in the stance phase and a marked vertical limp is present. The longer the lesion has been present, the less obvious the gait distortion becomes as the lumbo-pelvic-hip complex rapidly compensates in order to preserve energy.

On habitual movement testing, marked intra-pelvic torsion is noted on the forward/backward bending tests in standing and sitting, the ability to laterally translate the pelvic girdle is unilaterally blocked and the ipsilateral kinetic test in prone lying is severely limited.

On mobility testing, the innominate bone with the lesion is positioned in flexion/lateral rotation relative to the innominate bone of the opposite side. The L5 vertebra as well as the sacrum tends to be rotated towards the dysfunctional innominate bone. Passive extension/medial rotation of the innominate bone is restricted. The lesion occurs more frequently on the left side.

Extended/medially rotated innominate bone (anteriorly rotated/inflared)

Subjective findings. The mode of onset is usually insidious and the cause difficult to identify. The pain is usually diffuse throughout the lumbo-pelvic-hip complex with intermittent distal referral to the knee. Localization of the pain to the sacroiliac joint is rare. The aggravating activities are inconsistent and variable from day to day and the patient is often confused by their inability to depict a consistent pattern of pain behavior.

Objective findings. The patient's gait pattern is subtly altered by a shortened swing phase. Postural analysis reveals a multisegmental, thoracolumbar rotoscoliosis although the presence of a spinal curve is not pathognomonic of this lesion.

On habitual movement testing, intra-pelvic torsion is noted on the forward/backward bending tests in standing and sitting, the ability to laterally translate the pelvic girdle is unilaterally reduced and the ipsilateral kinetic test in standing is limited though not entirely blocked.

On mobility testing, the innominate bone with the lesion is positioned in extension/medial rotation relative to the innominate bone of the opposite side. The L5 vertebra as well as the sacrum tends to be rotated away from the dysfunctional innominate bone. Passive flexion/lateral rotation of the innominate bone is reduced. This lesion occurs more frequently on the right side and often in conjunction with other areas of restriction.

Superiorly subluxed/extended (flexed) innominate bone[36,37]

Subjective findings. The mode of onset is always traumatic although the event may not be recent. The characteristic etiology is a fall on the buttocks. The relationship between the vertical force and the axis of innominate extension/flexion dictates the degree of extension/flexion associated with the superior subluxation.[38] For example, if the vertical force occurs posterior to the paracoronal axis of extension/flexion (Fig. 9.1), the innominate bone is forced into extension (anterior rotation) as it subluxes in a superior direction. If the vertical force occurs anterior to the paracoronal axis of extension/flexion (Fig. 9.2), the innominate bone is forced into flexion (posterior rotation) as it subluxes in a superior direction.

The pain may be acute or chronic depending upon the stage of pathology and may be localized to the sacroiliac joint and/or distally referred to the knee. Over the long term, secondary decompensation of the lumbosacral junction can occur with concomitant pain

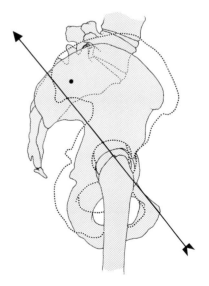

Fig. 9.1 The innominate bone will sublux superiorly and extend/anteriorly rotate (heavy dotted line) if the vertical force occurs posterior to the paracoronal axis of extension/flexion (dot).

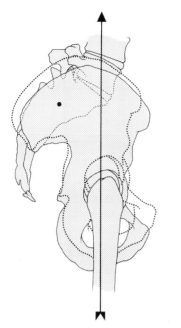

Fig. 9.2 The innominate bone will sublux superiorly and flex/posteriorly rotate (heavy dotted line) if the vertical force occurs anterior to the paracoronal axis of extension/flexion (dot).

and dysaesthesia depending upon the degree of degeneration (see Ch. 8). Coccygodynia secondary to the altered pull of the sacrospinous ligament is a common complaint.

Objective findings. On habitual movement testing, marked intra-pelvic torsion is noted on both the forward and backward bending tests in standing and sitting, the ability to laterally translate the pelvic girdle is unilaterally blocked and the ipsilateral kinetic tests in both standing and prone lying are limited.

On mobility testing, the innominate bone with the lesion is positioned superiorly and either flexed or extended relative to the innominate bone of the opposite side. The positional findings of the L5 vertebra and the sacrum are dictated by the flexion/extension component of the innominate distortion (see above). The tension of the sacrotuberous ligament is markedly reduced when the superior subluxation occurs in extension. When the subluxation occurs in conjunction with flexion of the innominate bone, the tension of the sacrotuberous ligament can be normal since the

flexion component of the lesion actually attenuates the ligament. Marked restriction of passive extension/flexion of the innominate bone is noted. The superiorly subluxed/extended lesion is commonly seen on the right whereas the superiorly subluxed/flexed lesion is commonly seen on the left.

Unilateral sacral flexion

Subjective findings. The mode of onset is usually traumatic. Commonly, the patient reports a lifting/twisting episode associated with a sudden twinge of pain localized to the sacroiliac joint. With time, the pain increases in both intensity and location to the point where attention is sought. The lift usually occurs in the absence of a pelvic tilt and therefore the sacrum has not been 'locked' between the innominate bones at the time of compression loading (see Ch. 5).

This lesion is also frequently seen in drivers involved in rear-end collisions. Typically, the patient had been wearing a three-point seatbelt and had the right foot firmly planted on the brake at the time of the impact. Initially, these patients present with an acute cervical whiplash and rarely complain of low back pain; however, as the cervical symptoms subside, the low back pain becomes evident.

The pain is dull, diffuse and rarely localized. Occipital headache is frequently reported in conjunction with this lesion and only resolves when the lumbo-pelvic-hip function has been restored.

Objective findings. On habitual movement testing, intra-pelvic torsion is noted during the forward bending test in standing, but may be minimal. The distortion becomes magnified when the test is repeated in sitting and often the multisegmental compensatory rotoscoliosis of the thoracolumbar spine is more prevalent. The ability to laterally translate the pelvic girdle is only minimally limited; however, the ipsilateral kinetic test in standing is reduced.

On mobility testing, the sacrum is positioned in unilateral flexion (i.e. a deep sacral sulcus together with an anterior sacral base and a posterior inferior lateral angle *on the same side*) in all three positions of the trunk—hyperflexion, hyperextension and neutral. Marked restriction of passive unilateral sacral extension is noted in all three positions.

Sacral torsion[37]

Subjective findings. The mode of onset may be either insidious or traumatic. The location of pain is variable, occasionally localized to the sacroiliac joint but not consistently. Frequently, the patient reports a very tender trigger point deep in the buttock, often within the piriformis muscle.

Objective findings. On habitual movement testing, intra-pelvic torsion is noted on either the forward or the backward bending tests in both standing and sitting. The distortion produces a multisegmental rotoscoliosis of the thoracolumbar spine. The ability to laterally translate the pelvic girdle is unilaterally restricted and the ipsilateral kinetic tests in both standing and prone lying are limited.

On mobility testing, the sacrum is positioned in rotation (i.e. a deep sacral sulcus together with an anterior sacral base on one side and a posterior inferior lateral angle *on the opposite side*) in one position of the trunk—hyperflexion or hyperextension. Passive unilateral sacral rotation is reduced in the direction opposite to that in which the bone is held.

This lesion is frequently seen in association with hypomobile disorders of the lumbosacral junction. If the L5 vertebra should be forced to rotate contrary to the sacrum when the injury occurs and subsequently becomes fixed in this position by muscle spasm, the patient presents with a very acutely distorted lumbo-pelvic region.[37,99] Positional testing of the L5 vertebra and the sacrum quickly reveals the disorder.

Treatment of the hypomobile pelvic girdle

History

At the turn of this century, sacroiliac joint dysfunction was treated in one of two ways—manipulation or immobilization.[4,38,42,83,142] The manipulation techniques for the 'subluxed' sacroiliac joints are poorly described in the literature and usually include non-specific pressure over the sacrum. Often the means of 'reduction' was quite gymnastic.

> The correction of the subluxation may be brought about in several ways. At times simply hyperextending the spine considerably by having the patient lie with a firm pillow under the 'hollow of the back', may, by raising the lumbar spine, draw the sacrum into place. At other times the same thing may be accomplished by having the patient lie face downward with the thighs and legs supported upon one table, the head and shoulders upon another, the body hanging entirely unsupported between. In this position the weight of the body drags the spine forward, which favors the replacement of the sacrum. If this is successful the plaster jacket which is to hold the spine and the pelvic joints may be applied before the patient is moved.[42]

Essentially, treatment of lumbo-pelvic-hip disorders has remained unchanged. Hypomobile joints are mobilized whereas hypermobile joints are immobilized. It is hoped that the criteria for classification have become less empirical and the treatment more humane.

The goal of therapy is to restore the optimal lumbo-pelvic-hip biomechanics via passive and active mobilization techniques and exercise programs. The soft tissues about the pelvic girdle are treated according to the presenting stage of repair (i.e. substrate, fibroblastic, maturation) which has been covered in detail in Chapter 6 and outlined in Chapter 8 under treatment of the hypomobile lumbosacral junction and should not require repetition here. This section will outline the specific mobilization techniques used to restore the osteokinematic function of the innominate bone and/or sacrum when localized hypomobility had been determined.

The myofascial, postural and ergonomic components of therapy pertinent to the lumbo-pelvic-hip complex will be discussed in Chapter 11.

Flexed/laterally rotated innominate bone

Passive mobilization technique (Fig. 9.3). This lesion may be either articular or myofas-

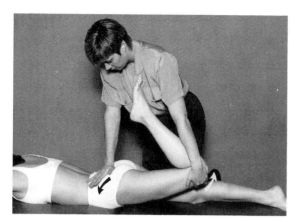

Fig. 9.3 Passive mobilization for the flexed/laterally rotated innominate bone (posteriorly rotated/outflared).

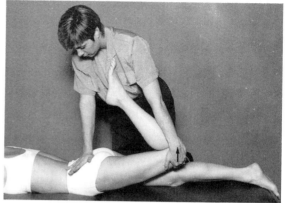

Fig. 9.4 Active mobilization for the flexed/laterally rotated innominate bone (posteriorly rotated/outflared). The arrow indicates the direction of resistance applied by the therapist.

cial in origin and in both instances the following technique, together with the active mobilization technique, is useful in restoring extension/medial rotation of the innominate bone. The technique can be graded in accordance with the irritability of the joint; however, if the lesion is articular in nature strong mobilization techniques (Grade 4[48]) are usually required to effect a change in the osteokinematic function.

With the patient prone, lying close to the edge of the table, the anterior aspect of the distal thigh is palpated with the caudal hand, while the PSIS of the innominate bone is palpated with the heel of the cranial hand.

The physiological limit of extension/medial rotation of the innominate bone is reached by passively extending the femur with the caudal hand and applying an anterolateral force to the innominate bone with the cranial hand. The passive mobilization is repeated by rhythmically extending the innominate bone with the two hands.

Active mobilization technique (Fig. 9.4). From the limit of the physiological range of extension/medial rotation of the innominate bone, the patient is instructed to resist further hip extension which is gently increased by the therapist. The isometric contraction is held for up to five seconds followed by a period of complete relaxation. The innominate bone is then passively taken to the new physiological range of extension/medial rotation. The tech-

nique is repeated three times followed by re-evaluation of the osteokinematic function of the innominate bone.

Home exercise program. Unilateral hip extension exercises (see Fig. 8.8) in the prone position repeated six times, six times per day are given to augment the mobilization techniques.

Extended/medially rotated innominate bone

Passive mobilization technique (Fig. 9.5). This lesion may be either articular or myofas-

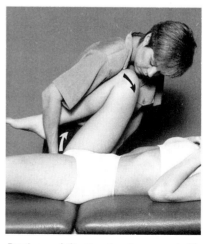

Fig. 9.5 Passive mobilization for the extended/medially rotated innominate bone (anteriorly rotated/inflared).

cial in origin and in both instances the following technique, together with the active mobilization technique, is useful in restoring flexion/lateral rotation of the innominate bone.

With the patient supine, lying close to the edge of the table, the ischial tuberosity is palpated with the caudal hand. The flexed hip and knee are supported against the therapist's caudal shoulder and arm. The anterior aspect of the ASIS and the innominate bone are palpated with the cranial hand.

The physiological limit of flexion/lateral rotation of the innominate bone is reached by passively flexing the femur with the caudal hand and applying a posteromedial force to the innominate bone with the cranial hand. The passive mobilization is repeated by rhythmically flexing the innominate bone with the two hands.

Active mobilization technique (Fig. 9.6). At the limit of the physiological range of flexion/lateral rotation of the innominate bone, the patient is instructed to resist further hip flexion which is gently increased by the therapist. The isometric contraction is held for up to five seconds, followed by a period of complete relaxation. The innominate bone is then passively taken to the new physiological

range of flexion/lateral rotation. The technique is repeated three times followed by re-evaluation of the osteokinematic function of the innominate bone.

Home exercise program. Unilateral hip flexion exercises (see Fig. 8.12) in the supine position repeated six times, six times per day are given to augment the mobilization techniques.

Superiorly subluxed/extended innominate bone

Passive mobilization technique (Fig. 9.7). This lesion is always articular in origin and requires a high velocity, low amplitude thrust technique for restoration of function of the innominate bone. The lumbosacral junction must be mobile before any reduction of the sacroiliac joint is attempted.

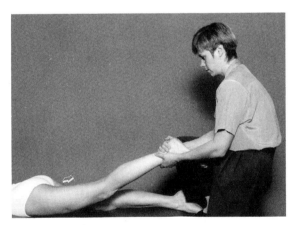

Fig. 9.7 Passive mobilization for the superiorly subluxed/extended innominate bone (upslip in anterior rotation).

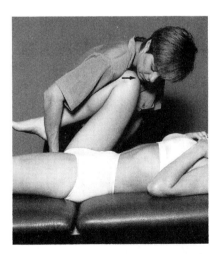

Fig. 9.6 Active mobilization for the extended/medially rotated innominate bone (anteriorly rotated/inflared). The arrow indicates the direction of resistance applied by the therapist.

With the patient lying prone, the lower extremity is grasped with both hands just proximal to the talocrural joint. The plane of the sacroiliac joint is located via a series of longitudinal pulls through the lower extremity in varying degrees of femoral abduction and extension. The femoral position which yields the greatest degree of inferior excursion of the lower extremity is sought. From this position, a gradual longitudinal pull is applied until the physiological limit of range has been reached. If this position is painless, a high velocity, low amplitude tug is applied through the leg to the sacroiliac joint. The success of the technique is evaluated by the immediate return of the osteokinematic function of the innominate bone.

The patient is advised to return for follow-up in two days during which time all activities involving vertical translation of the sacroiliac joint (i.e. jumping) should be avoided. There are no specific exercises required.

Superiorly subluxed/flexed innominate bone

Passive mobilization technique (Fig. 9.8). This lesion is always articular in origin and also requires a high velocity, low amplitude thrust technique for restoration of function of the innominate bone. The technique is identical to the one described for the superiorly subluxed/extended innominate bone with the following exceptions.

The patient is lying supine, and the plane of the sacroiliac joint is located via a series of longitudinal pulls through the lower extremity in varying degrees of femoral abduction and flexion. Again, the initial pull of the lower extremity should be painless. The success of the technique is also evaluated by the immediate return of the osteokinematic func-

tion of the innominate bone. The follow-up advice to the patient is the same.

Unilateral sacral flexion

Passive mobilization technique (Fig. 9.9). With the patient prone, lying close to the edge of the table, the anterior aspect of the distal thigh is palpated with the caudal hand while the cranial hand palpates the ipsilateral sacral sulcus. With the caudal hand, a longitudinal pull is applied to the lower extremity in varying degrees of femoral abduction until the plane of the sacroiliac joint is located. The femur is then medially rotated and gently supported via the therapist's knee.

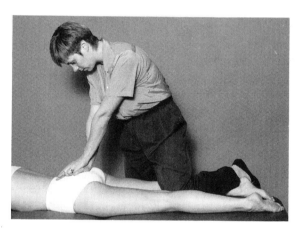

Fig. 9.9 Passive mobilization for the unilateral sacral flexion.

The inferior lateral angle of the sacrum (on the side of the sacral flexion) is palpated with the heel of the caudal hand, reinforced with the cranial hand. An anterosuperior force is applied to the inferior lateral angle in varying degrees of obliquity to determine the plane of the sacroiliac joint. The patient is then instructed to breathe in deeply for three breaths during which time the therapist continues to apply an anterosuperior force to the inferior lateral angle of the sacrum. The force is maintained during the expiratory phase as well. The mobilization is repeated three times followed by re-evaluation of the osteokinematic function of the sacrum.

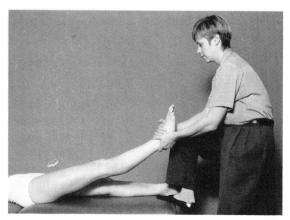

Fig. 9.8 Passive mobilization for the superiorly subluxed/flexed innominate bone (upslip in posterior rotation).

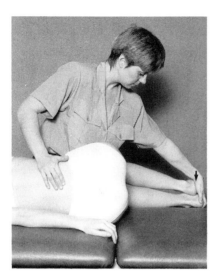

Fig. 9.10 Active mobilization for the left sacral torsion lesion evident in hyperflexion of the trunk. The arrow indicates the direction of resistance applied by the therapist.

Sacral torsion

The lumbosacral junction must be mobile prior to treating the sacral torsion lesion.

Active mobilization technique for the left sacral torsion lesion evident in hyperflexion of the trunk (Fig. 9.10). With the patient in left sidelying, the lower arm positioned behind the back and the upper arm hanging over the edge of the table, the interspinous space between the L5 vertebra and the sacrum is palpated with the cranial hand. The lower extremities are supported bilaterally by grasping the feet with the caudal hand. The hips and knees are comfortably flexed and supported on the therapist's abdomen. The lumbosacral junction should be in a neutral position, ensured by first flexing the articulation fully and then returning to neutral.

The physiological limit of sacral torsion is then reached by allowing the feet to descend towards the floor until a firm resistance is encountered. The patient is instructed to gently lift the feet from this position, towards the ceiling and to simultaneously reach towards the floor with the upper arm. The elevation of the lower extremities is resisted by the therapist and the isometric contraction

is maintained for up to five seconds, followed by a period of complete relaxation. The sacrum is then passively taken to the new physiological range of rotation by allowing the feet to descend further towards the floor. The technique is repeated three times followed by re-evaluation of the osteokinematic function of the sacrum.

Case history

A 25-year-old nurse presented at the clinic four days after the acute onset of left sacroiliac joint pain following a horizontal lift of a patient up the bed. The onset of the pain was very sudden but not severe enough to warrant immediate attention. Since spontaneous resolution was not occurring, she sought medical attention and was subsequently referred for evaluation and treatment. The location of the pain had spread to include the left posterior hemi-pelvis. Dysaesthesia was not reported. The aggravating factors included any prolonged activity.

Objectively, habitual movement testing revealed asymmetry of pelvic girdle motion in both forward and backward bending in both standing and sitting. Lateral translation of the pelvic girdle was limited to the right during left lateral bending of the trunk. The ipsilateral kinetic test in both standing and prone lying was restricted on the left.

Subsequent positional testing revealed a deep left sacral sulcus, an anterior left sacral base and a postero-inferior left inferior lateral angle. These findings were consistent in all three positions of the trunk—hyperflexion, neutral and hyperextension, Mobility testing of the sacrum revealed restricted extension and left rotation, again in all three positions of the trunk.

Tenderness of the left dorsal sacroiliac ligament was noted; however, arthrokinetic testing for pelvic girdle stability was normal.

This is a typical clinical presentation of an acute left sacral flexion lesion and resolved rapidly with the appropriate mobilization technique described above combined with electrotherapeutic analgesic modalities.

HYPERMOBILITY WITH OR WITHOUT PAIN

Hypermobility of the pelvic girdle can occur following repeated microtrauma, one major trauma or secondary to hormonal changes such as those associated with pregnancy (see Ch. 5). The essential objective finding for classification here is *increased* osteokinematic motion of either the sacrum or the innominate bone.

Subjective findings

The mode of onset is usually insidious. The patient reports a gradual onset of sacroiliac joint and/or pubic symphysis pain which may radiate into the buttock, posterior thigh and/or abdomen and groin. The aggravating activities commonly include:

1. unilateral weight-bearing
2. bending forward
3. lifting
4. lying supine and rolling over from this position
5. fast walking
6. any activity for prolonged periods of time.

Clicking of the pubic symphysis and/or sacroiliac joint is frequently reported.[53] Rest usually affords relief as long as the hypermobile joint is not under stress while in the resting position.

Objective findings

Mobility

Objectively, the hypermobile patient may adopt altered lumbo-pelvic-hip movement patterns to compensate for the loss of kinetic stability within the pelvic girdle. The typical gait pattern is one of excessive lateral shift of the center of gravity with each stance phase, somewhat like a waddling duck. As with lumbosacral hypermobility, forward flexion is achieved by walking the hands down the thighs and back up to return to erect standing. If the pelvic girdle is manually stabilized (Fig. 9.11) and the patient is instructed to repeat the forward bend test, he/she is able to do so more freely and with less pain.[42,116]

Specific mobility testing of the pelvic girdle reveals increased flexion/extension of the innominate bone at the pubic symphysis. According to Young,[142] hypermobility of the pubic symphysis can only occur if the sacroiliac joint has also lost kinetic stability. Bellamy notes that 'The most reliable clinical sign of instability of disruption of the SI joint is that of disruption of the pubic symphysis. This will only occur when there is excessive movement at the SI joint and can be readily assessed by

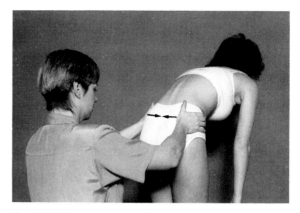

Fig. 9.11 Transverse manual stabilization of the pelvic girdle will improve both the quantity and the quality of forward bending of the trunk when hypermobility is present.

observing the relative movements of the pubic rami on weight bearing alternately on either leg'.[10]

Stability

The transverse anterior and the superoinferior pubic symphysis stress tests are usually painful in the pathological hypermobile patient. The strength of the dorsal sacroiliac ligaments is so great (see Ch. 4) that it is doubtful that a painful transverse posterior stress test is indicative of attenuation of these ligaments. Since the test also compresses the anterior aspect of the sacroiliac joint, it is more likely that pain produced during this test is intra-articular in origin.

Treatment of the hypermobile pelvic girdle

History

Immobilization was, and still is, the treatment of choice for hypermobile joints. At the turn of this century, the means of immobilization for the pelvic girdle included:

1. a two-inch band of plaster applied just below the ASISs encircling the pelvis and reapplied weekly for four weeks followed by the application of a four-inch elastic webbing belt which was to be worn indefinitely[4]

2. a plaster jacket which encircled the pelvis and extended unilaterally down the leg to the knee, worn for four months, followed by a shorter plaster jacket worn for an additional two months which was subsequently replaced by a light pelvic belt.[83]

Hypermobility during pregnancy was widely recognized and treated postpartum via immobilization.

> It is the state or condition of the pelvic joints, rather than the state of the woman's general health which should determine the date of her rising after childbirth . . . . [and] should vary directly with the size of the foetal head and inversely with the size of the woman's pelvis. That is to say if the child is of large size or born with a great degree of moulding of the head, the woman should be kept in the prone position for a longer period than the stipulated ten days or so in which in the hurry and bustle of modern life is all that is allowed to her.[19]

Present-day treatment

The loss of kinetic stability within the pelvic girdle is a challenge to treat and, if successful, the rewards are great since instability can be very debilitating. The treatment given follows the principles of wound repair outlined in the

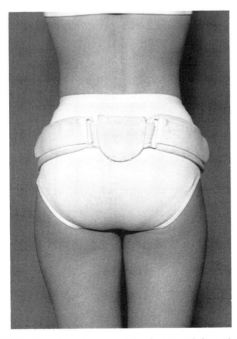

Fig. 9.12 An external support for hypermobility of the pelvic girdle.

treatment of the hypermobile lumbosacral junction. The temporary application of an external support (Fig. 9.12) can be very helpful during all three stages of repair.[41] The support should be worn at all times when weight-bearing. Initially, a seven-day trial period is required to assess the success of the external stabilization. If the patient's pain is increased during the trial period, the use of the support should be abandoned. As with all rehabilitation of the lumbo-pelvic-hip complex, myofascial, postural and ergonomic training should be an integral part of the treatment (see Ch. 11).

If the degree of trauma and the subsequent kinetic decompensation results in a permanent loss of pelvic girdle kinetic strength, a sclerosing injection of the dorsal sacroiliac ligaments may be indicated.[116] Alternately, the unstable sacroiliac joint may be surgically arthrodesed.[116]

Case history

A 24-year-old stenographer presented with sacral pain which had developed insidiously over the past three weeks. The patient was 28 weeks' pregnant at the time of examination.

The pain was sharp and local to the right sacroiliac joint as well as dull and diffuse over the entire aspect of the sacrum. The sharp pain was aggravated by supine lying, rolling over in bed and unilateral weight-bearing through the right leg. The dull pain was particularly aggravated by walking. A mild discomfort was also noted centrally at the pubic symphysis.

Objectively, forward bending of the trunk was possible, though painful, and required extensive support of the body weight with the hands on the thighs. When compression was applied transversely through the pelvic girdle, forward bending was achieved with a significant reduction in pain.

Mobility testing revealed slight hypermobility of both sacroiliac joints and excessive superoinferior mobility of the pubic symphysis. The transverse anterior and the superoinferior pubic symphysis arthrokinetic tests were painful. Baer's point was extremely tender to palpation on the right.

This is a common clinical presentation of hypermobility secondary to pregnancy and represents an arthrokinetic decompensation of the pelvic girdle. An external support was prescribed, which afforded moderate relief, and was worn for the duration of the pregnancy as well as the early postpartum recovery period. With time, the kinetic stability of the pelvic girdle returned and the patient was able to discontinue the use of the support and return to her previous level of function.

NORMAL MOBILITY WITH PAIN

Patients presenting with localized pain within the pelvic girdle in the absence of 'hard' objective findings are a challenge to treat. Clinically, several mobility tests reproduce the pain but never consistently. Careful objective evaluation of mobility reveals normal function. As with the lumbosacral junction, the only cause of a biomechanical nature for this dysfunction can be overuse of the articular and myofascial tissues secondary to altered function elsewhere. A complete postural analysis is required at this stage if rehabilitation is to be successful. A global approach to assessment and treatment is often the only means of improving function with these patients. Alternately, the patient may have a disorder which is not biomechanical in nature (see Table 9.1), a possibility of which the clinician must always be aware.

10

The hip: clinical syndromes

CLASSIFICATION

Disorders of the hip are not rare; however, early detection is often difficult. Primary degenerative arthrosis can occur very early at this articulation. Grieve has noted that 'about 10% to 11% of people aged below 30 years have a degree of arthrosis, some with hip involvement'.[49] Slight restriction of motion at this joint can produce dramatic compensatory effects at both the sacroiliac joint and the lumbosacral junction. The subsequent decompensation of the lumbo-pelvic region can only be resolved by restoring the mobility of the hip.

Hip disorders are commonly categorized according to the age group in which they occur (Table 10.1). Alternately, the disorders have been classified as articular or non-articular (Table 10.2).

For the clinical manual therapist, classifications which follow a biomechanical model based on mobility, bearing in mind the specific disorders relative to the patient's age group, continue to prove more useful in facilitating a consistent approach to assessment and treatment. In keeping with this model, disorders of the hip region can be classified into two groups, each of which describes the objective findings noted on mobility testing. They include:
1. Hypomobility with or without pain
2. Normal mobility with pain.

This classification pertains to the presence

121

Table 10.1 Classification of hip disorders according to age group[24]

Newborn
Congenital dislocation of the hip

Ages 4–12 years
Perthe's disease
Tuberculosis
Transitory arthritis

Ages12–17 Years
Slipped femoral epiphysis
Osteochondritis dissecans

Young adults
Muscle lesions
Bursitis

Adults
Arthritis
  Osteoarthritis
  Rheumatoid arthritis
  Ankylosing spondylitis
Bursitis
Loose bodies

Table 10.2 Articular v. non-articular disorders of the hip[2]

Articular disorders of the hip
Congenital deformities
  Congenital dislocation of the hip
Arthritis
  Transient arthritis of children
  Pyogenic arthritis
  Rheumatoid arthritis
  Tuberculous arthritis
  Osteoarthritis
  Ankylosing spondylitis
Osteochondritis
  Perthes' disease (pseudocoxalgia)
Mechanical disorders
  Slipped upper femoral epiphysis
  Osteitis deformans (Paget's disease)

Non-articular disorders in the region of the hip
Deformities
  Coxa vara
Infections
  Tuberculosis of the trochanteric bursa

or absence of osteokinematic function of the femur relative to the innominate bone and is directly dependent upon the composite arthrokinematic and myokinematic function of the hip. Like the lumbosacral junction and the pelvic girdle, this classification does not provide a specific anatomical or physiological cause for the aberrant mobility noted; however, it is important to recall that the goal of

therapy is to improve functional movement patterns regardless of the underlying diagnosis. The aim of all evaluation procedures is to identify the system (i.e. articular v. myofascial) which is aberrantly altering the osteokinematic function of the femur/innominate bones during functional movement so that treatment can be directed accordingly.

HYPOMOBILITY WITH OR WITHOUT PAIN

The hip joint, like all other synovial joints, deteriorates slowly and consequently can present a variety of clinical pictures. In the early stages of pathology, altered afferent input from the mechanoreceptors within the joint capsule (see Ch. 4) can adversely affect the perceptual component of static joint position, dynamic proprioception and kinetic stability as well as the resting tone of the postural muscles about the hip joint. The patient may state that the limb feels weak rather than restricted in range, particularly during athletic endeavors.

'The implications are obvious—if degenerative change has grossly disturbed afferent impulse traffic from capsular mechanoreceptors, the partial loss of the 'governor' for joint congruity has increased the susceptibility of such joints to articular strains from normally trivial stress'.[49] Thus the degenerative process is facilitated and the articular restriction is slowly manifested.

The essential objective finding for classification here is *decreased* osteokinematic motion of the femur relative to the innominate bone. The etiology may be either articular or myofascial and is not necessarily restricted to older individuals.

Subjective findings

The mode of onset is usually insidious although trauma can certainly be a factor. The location of pain is highly variable and often confusing, notably when decompensation of the lumbo-pelvic region has occurred in conjunction with the hip disorder. Wroblewski[49,139] studied the pain patterns in 89 patients with osteoarthritis of the hip joint and the variety of presentation noted is tabulated in Table 10.3. The hip joint, being derived from the L3 mesoderm, can refer pain anywhere within the L3 dermatome and/or sclerotome. Clinically, it is common to find the primary complaint being *knee* pain which the patient completely dissociates from 'the usual backache' and often denies local hip pain entirely.

Table 10.3 Pain patterns in 89 patients with osteoarthritis of the hip joint (From Wroblewski)[49,139]

Area of pain	Number of patients
Greater trochanter	71
Medial buttock	40
Groin	47
Anterior thigh	63
Knee	70
Shin	40

With moderate articular degeneration, the aggravating activities include walking, stair climbing/descent and weight-bearing in flexion (i.e. squat). In the early stages, more demanding activities such as sport may be required to aggravate the condition.

Objective findings

Gait

Hypomobility of the hip is reflected in the patient's gait pattern. The stance phase is often shortened, thus creating a vertical limp. If the aberrant mechanoreceptor input from the articular capsule significantly alters the myokinetic function (i.e. decreased gluteal strength), there may also be a loss of arthrokinetic dynamic stability compensated for by a lateral limp. The center of gravity deviates laterally in order to reduce the myokinetic requirements of unilateral stance (see Ch. 5). The degree to which the vertical and lateral limp are exhibited depends upon the degree of loss of range of motion and kinaesthesis at the hip.

Mobility

The tests of habitual movement in weight-bearing will reflect even a minor limitation of motion at the hip. The pattern of restricted motion is dependent upon the underlying etiology (i.e. articular v. myofascial). The forward/backward bending tests, lateral bending tests and striding tests may all be adversely affected by the restriction. Alterations from the normal biomechanics should alert the examiner to a more detailed examination.

The osteokinematic tests of physiological mobility disclose the pattern of restriction which can be either capsular or non-capsular in origin.[24] The fully established capsular pattern of restriction of the hip joint is:
1. 50°–55° limitation of femoral abduction
2. 0° of femoral medial rotation from neutral
3. 90° limitation of femoral flexion
4. 10°–30° limitation of femoral extension
5. femoral lateral rotation and adduction is fully maintained.

However, as was previously mentioned, the degenerative process of the hip joint occurs over time such that, in the presence of early pathology, the only objective finding may be a slight limitation of medial rotation and flexion. As the pathology progresses, the full capsular pattern of restriction emerges.

The quadrant test is universally affected when the joint is hypomobile.[49] Often, a painful 'bump' can be palpated during the flexion/adduction phase of the test associated with muscular resistance (hypertonicity) and reactive spasm if the joint is irritable.

The end feel of motion during mobility testing primarily differentiates the articular restriction from the myofascial. A very hard end feel is indicative of an articular restriction whereas a softer end feel is indicative of a myofascial restriction. Clinically, the two are usually seen in combination given the intimate articular neuromuscular physiology.

The arthrokinematics of the hip joint are relatively limited in comparison to the gross physiological movements they facilitate. If, however, arthrokinematic testing reveals decreased mobility in the presence of decreased osteokinematic function, an articular restriction is confirmed. Emphasis should be placed on the quality of movement as opposed to the quantity of movement for differential diagnosis.

Stability

The tests for static arthrokinetic stability (i.e. ligament stress tests) are normal in the hypomobile group. Proprioception and *dynamic* stability, however, are often deficient due to the altered neurophysiology.

Muscle function—myokinematics

Janda[56,57,58] has observed that very early in the degenerative process of the hip joint certain muscle groups respond by tightening (postural muscles) while others respond by weakening (phasic muscles). This alteration in function can certainly contribute to the chronic imbalance of functional movement patterns and ultimately the decompensation of the lumbo-pelvic-hip region (see also Ch. 9).

To review, the postural muscles relative to the hip which tend to tighten include the:

1. hamstrings—limitation of femoral flexion when the ipsilateral knee is extended
2. rectus femoris—limitation of femoral extension when the knee is flexed
3. iliopsoas—limitation of femoral extension/medial rotation
4. tensor fascia lata—limitation of femoral adduction/lateral rotation
5. adductors—limitation of femoral abduction
6. piriformis—limitation of femoral medial rotation when the femur is less than 60° flexed, and of lateral rotation/adduction when the femur is greater than 60° flexed.

The phasic muscles which tend to weaken include the:

1. gluteus maximus, medius, minimus
2. vasti muscles.

'The inhibitory effect of a tight postural muscle is evidenced when weakness of the gluteus maximus accompanies tightness of the iliopsoas. Hip extension is slightly abnormal, lumbar lordosis tends to increase and abnormal loading of the lumbo-sacral segment initiates chronic changes which can be a cause of pain, in both low back and hip'.[49]

Sign of the buttock

According to Cyriax, all major lesions or serious pathology in the buttock present with 'an arresting pattern of physical signs that draws immediate attention to the buttock. Passive hip flexion with the knee held extended . . . is slightly limited and painful. Passive hip flexion, this time with the knee flexed too, is again limited and more painful. Further examination reveals a non-capsular pattern of limitation of movement at the hip joint'.[24] The end feel of motion is empty (i.e. limited by pain) as opposed to that of articular or myofascial tissue resistance.

This sign should alert the examiner to the potential presence of serious pathology such as:

1. osteomyelitis of the upper femur
2. chronic septic sacroiliac arthritis
3. ischiorectal abscess
4. septic bursitis
5. rheumatic fever with bursitis
6. neoplasm at the upper femur
7. iliac neoplasm
8. fractured sacrum.

If the 'sign of the buttock' is manifested during the examination, the presence/absence of serious pathology should be confirmed prior to initiating treatment.

Treatment of the hypomobile hip joint

Treatment of the hip joint forms part of the overall rehabilitation of the lumbo-pelvic-hip complex. To review, the ultimate goal is to restore the optimal function of the entire unit both kinematically as well as kinetically. The following section outlines the specific therapy indicated during each stage of repair (i.e. substrate, fibroblastic, maturation) when localized hypomobility of the hip joint is found.

The myofascial, postural and ergonomic components of therapy pertinent to the lumbo-pelvic-hip complex will be discussed in Chapter 11.

Substrate phase

During the first four to six days after injury the goal of treatment is hemostasis of the wound. At home, the frequent application of ice together with rest is the treatment of choice.

At the clinic, electrotherapeutic analgesic modalities such as transcutaneous nerve stimulation and interferential current therapy can afford relief from pain; however, the patient should not attend at this stage if the physical stresses induced are greater than the relief gained.

Fibroblastic phase

With the resolution of active range of movement, the osteokinematic restriction becomes apparent. If the pattern of restriction is capsular, the joint is implicated as the etiological factor. If the pattern of restriction is non-capsular, the extra-articular tissues are implicated as the etiological factor. With respect to the articular tissues, the goal of treatment during this stage of repair is primarily to restore mobility. Passive and active mobilization techniques are utilized to restore the articular kinematics combined with a specific home exercise program.

Distraction—passive mobilization technique (Fig. 10.1). This is an extremely useful preliminary mobilization technique which can be graded according to the irritability of the joint. Initially, gentle grades are indicated, keeping well within the range of pain and reactive muscle spasm. The large afferent fiber input from the Type I and II mechanoreceptors located in the articular capsule inhibits the centripetal transmission of the small fiber input (nociception) at the spinal cord, thus reducing the perception of pain via the spinal gating mechanism (see Ch. 4).

With the patient lying supine, the proximal thigh is palpated while the distal leg rests over the therapist's shoulder. The joint is distracted by applying a distolateral force parallel to the

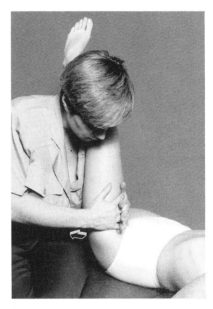

Fig. 10.1 Passive mobilization of the hip joint—distraction.

neck of the femur. The posteroanterior orientation of the applied force will vary depending upon the degree of femoral anteversion present.

Inferior glide—passive mobilization technique (Fig. 10.2). With the patient lying supine, the proximal thigh is palpated. An inferior femoral glide is induced by applying an inferolateral force along the longitudinal axis of the femur. This technique is also graded in

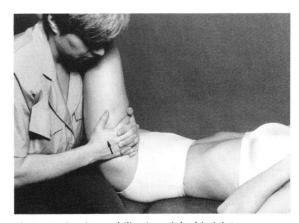

Fig. 10.2 Passive mobilization of the hip joint—inferior glide for the restoration of femoral abduction.

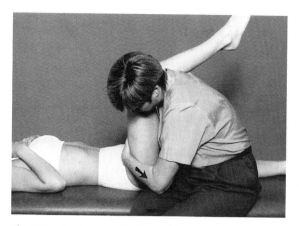

Fig. 10.3 Passive mobilization of the hip joint—posterolateral/anteromedial glide for the restoration of femoral medial/lateral rotation.

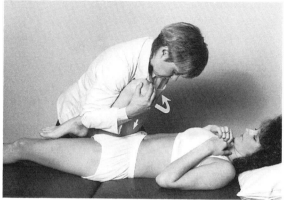

Fig. 10.4 Passive mobilization of the joint hip—quadrant technique.

accordance with the·irritability of the joint. The neurophysiological effects have been described above. Arthrokinematically, the technique attempts to restore the glide associated with the osteokinematic motion of femoral abduction.

Posteroanterior glide—passive mobilization technique (Fig. 10.3). With the patient lying supine, the proximal thigh is palpated. A posteroanterior glide is induced by applying a posterolateral/anteromedial force parallel to the plane of the acetabular fossa.

The technique is graded according to the level of joint irritability and is utilized to restore the arthrokinematic glide associated with the osteokinematic motion of medial/lateral femoral rotation.

Quadrant technique—passive mobilization technique (Fig. 10.4). With the patient lying supine, the flexed knee of the lower extremity is palpated with the caudal hand. The anterior aspect of the iliac crest and the anterior superior iliac spine are palpated with the cranial hand. The femur is passively flexed, adducted, medially rotated and longitudinally compressed to scour the inner aspect of the joint. From this position, the femur is taken into abduction and lateral rotation while maintaining the degree of femoral flexion. By repetitively scouring the various painful 'bumps and lumps' palpable within the hip joint, the

osteokinematic function of the femur can be effectively restored.

Active mobilization technique (Fig. 10.5). The hip joint can be actively mobilized via the myofascial system in the following manner. The femur is initially taken to the limit of the available range of motion (i.e. flexion/medial rotation). The patient is instructed to resist further motion from this position while the therapist attempts to increase the range (in

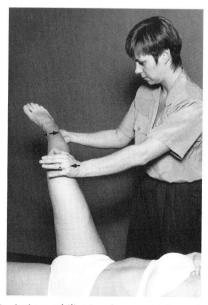

Fig. 10.5 Active mobilization for a restriction of femoral flexion/medial rotation. The arrows indicate the direction of resistance applied by the therapist.

the direction of the restriction). This is not a tug-of-war but rather a gentle isometric contraction which is held for up to five seconds followed by a period of complete relaxation. The femur is then passively taken to the new physiological range of motion and the technique repeated as often as progress occurs.

The restoration of optimal femoral function ultimately requires attention to both the articular and the neuromuscular system; thus there is need for integrated neuromuscular techniques such as proprioceptive neuromuscular facilitation techniques which should not need description here.

Home exercise program. Range of motion exercises which are directed towards resolving the individual's specific pattern of restriction are indicated at this stage of repair. If unilateral weight-bearing is still painful, all weight-bearing exercises should be avoided and swimming encouraged instead.

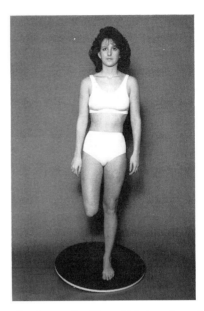

Fig. 10.6 The foot and ankle wobble board requires weight-bearing, precision balance and co-ordination and is a useful exercise modality for neuromuscular re-education of the lumbo-pelvic-hip complex.

Maturation phase

Mobilization techniques. If restrictive capsular adhesions have developed during the fibroblastic stage of repair, stronger passive mobilization techniques will be required to restore the optimal kinematic function of the hip joint. The active and passive mobilization techniques utilized at this stage of repair are identical to those previously described except that the joint is taken strongly and specifically to the physiological limit of range (Grade 4).

Home exercise program. The specific exercise given at this stage should be designed to restore not only the range of femoral motion, but the arthrokinetic stability at the hip joint, both static (weight-bearing) and dynamic (proprioceptive function). The balance board (Fig. 10.6) is a very useful exercise tool since it requires weight-bearing, precision balance and co-ordination. The exercises can be progressed from very easy to extremely difficult by increasing the diameter of the hemisphere upon which the board is attached. As well, exercises for global lumbo-pelvic-hip function should be included.

NORMAL MOBILITY WITH PAIN

The presence of normal mobility at the hip joint associated with pain may be indicative of:

1. a mild inflammatory intra-articular process secondary to trauma and/or overuse of the articular and myofascial tissues in compensation for altered function elsewhere
2. an isolated ligament sprain following an athletic injury and/or other major trauma
3. a muscle sprain following an athletic injury and/or other major trauma
4. an inflamed bursa (iliopsoas, gluteal, ischial, trochanteric).

Traumatic arthritis

A mild inflammatory intra-articular process (mild traumatic arthritis) is painful but does not restrict the range of motion at the hip joint. Although walking aggravates the symptoms, the gait pattern is within normal limits. The specific mobility tests which reproduce the pain are consistent with those that are restricted in the capsular pattern (i.e. medial rotation and flexion). Compression of the joint is painful whereas distraction affords relief.

The arthrokinematic tests are normal as are the tests for myokinematic function. In the absence of any known trauma, the etiology of decompensation may lie extrinsic to the hip joint itself.

Ligament sprains

Isolated ligament sprains of this joint are rare in clinical practice. The major ligaments about the hip joint are among the strongest in the body and a fracture will usually occur before the ligament is sprained. Rarely, an isolated ligament injury occurs in combination with a myofascial sprain following a major traumatic incident which rapidly takes the joint beyond its normal range. The sports in which such injuries can occur are those which demand excessive articular mobility including gymnastics, dancing and the martial arts as well as those in which excessive trauma is easily encountered such as soccer, skiing, football and ice skating.

The location of pain is usually specific to the damaged tissue and aggravated by the osteokinematic and arthrokinetic tests which stress them (see Ch. 7). If the hip joint is restricted by the lesion, the pattern of restriction is noncapsular. In the acute injury, the resisted tests of myokinematic function may also be painful if the muscle being tested pulls on the lesioned ligament.

Muscle sprains

Contractile tissue lesions (i.e. muscle sprains) about the hip are commonly seen in athletes. The degree of injury is dependent upon the extent of trauma encountered. The mode of onset is definitely traumatic and the individual usually reports a 'snapping' sensation at the time of injury. If the injury is major, a tense haematoma rapidly develops at the wound site. In minor injuries, the onset may be insidious over a longer period of time and not necessarily accompanied by a haematoma. The location of pain is localized to the damaged tissue and aggravated by the specific mobility tests which stress the lesioned tissue. The pattern of restriction, if any, is noncapsular.

The resisted tests of myokinematic function are consistently painful when the lesioned tissue is recruited. The specific muscles commonly injured include the rectus femoris, the hamstrings and the adductor muscles.

Bursitis

Bursitis about the hip joint is not rare. Acute bursitis is extremely painful, with most motions of the joint being restricted by pain as opposed to muscle or capsular tissue (i.e. the end feel is empty). The resisted tests of myokinematic function are also painful since they invariably squeeze the inflamed bursa. The condition is self-limiting in ten days to three weeks.

Chronic bursitis is more difficult to diagnose in that the pattern of clinical presentation is often inconsistent. The location of pain is variable, the mode of onset usually insidious and the aggravating factors rarely consistent. That some things hurt some of the time and others hurt at other times is a familiar history. The mobility tests are inconsistently painful. Resisted tests often reproduce the pain, again inconsistently. The end feel of motion is soft, as opposed to empty, but may be hard if an underlying arthritic condition coexists.

Treatment

The treatment required for these soft tissue lesions in the varying stages of repair (substrate, fibroblastic, maturation) has been outlined in detail in Chapter 6.

11

Muscles, posture and ergonomics

The successful rehabilitation of the lumbo-pelvic-hip complex requires the restoration of efficient myofascial and postural function. In addition, the employment of optimal static and dynamic ergonomics (i.e. sitting and standing postures, walking and lifting biomechanics) is essential if a recurrence is to be prevented. Following the restoration of articular function within the lumbo-pelvic-hip complex, attention should be directed towards the postural and/or phasic muscles which tend to tighten and/or weaken since the abnormal movement patterns they induce may persist long after the articular function has been restored.

POSTURAL MUSCLES

Relative to the pelvic girdle, the postural muscles which tend to tighten include the:
1. erector spinae/quadratus lumborum
2. hamstrings
3. rectus femoris
4. iliopsoas
5. tensor fascia lata
6. adductors
7. piriformis.
   Clinically, the tight postural muscles exhibit a restriction or deviation of habitual movement *in the presence of normal articular mobility.* The treatment includes active mobilization techniques combined with a specific home exercise program designed to restore the optimal length of the muscle.

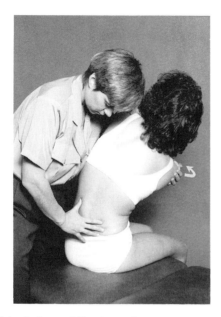

Fig. 11.1 Active mobilization technique for stretching the spinal extensor muscles.

Erector spinae/quadratus lumborum

Active mobilization technique (Fig. 11.1)

With the patient sitting, feet supported, arms crossed and the vertebral column in a neutral position, the contralateral shoulder is palpated with the ventral arm. The ipsilateral erector spinae/quadratus lumborum muscle group is stretched by laterally bending the patient away from and rotating the patient towards the therapist to the limit of the physiological range of motion. The myofascia on the side of the produced convexity should now be on stretch.

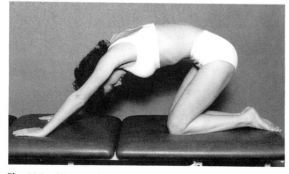

Fig. 11.2 Home exercise program for stretching the spinal extensor muscles.

The patient is instructed to hold this position while the therapist attempts to further increase the lateral bend/rotation components of the stretch. The contraction may be either isometric or eccentric and is held for up to five seconds followed by a period of complete relaxation. The thoraco-lumbar spine is taken to the limit of the new physiological range of motion and the technique repeated from this point.

Home exercise program (Fig. 11.2)

The patient is instructed to start from the four-point kneeling position, and to flex the thoracolumbar spine by kyphosing in a posterior direction. While maintaining this kyphosis, the patient is to sit back on the heels, without displacing the hands, until moderate stretch of the spinal extensors is perceived. This position is maintained for 30 seconds to 1 minute followed by a return to the four-point kneeling position. The stretch is repeated as often as possible during the day with the minimum being six stretches, six times per day.

Alternately, the myofascia may be stretched unilaterally from the four-point kneeling position. The patient is instructed to flex the thoracolumbar spine by kyphosing in a posterior direction, followed by lateral bending of the trunk away from the tight muscle group. The position is maintained for 30 seconds to 1 minute followed by a return to the four-point kneeling position. The stretch is repeated as often as possible during the day with the minimum being six stretches, six times per day.

Hamstrings

Active mobilization (Fig. 11.3)

With the patient lying supine, the lower extremity is palpated above the ankle. While maintaining the knee in extension, the femur is flexed at the hip joint. The therapist's cranial hand monitors any subsequent flexion of the innominate bone via the anterior aspect of the

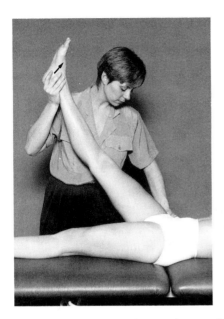

Fig. 11.3 Active mobilization technique for stretching the hamstring muscles.

hamstring muscle group while maintaining the vertebral column in a neutral position and the knee joint in full extension. The patient is instructed to start from this position and to forward bend the *pelvic girdle on the femur*, not the vertebral column, until a moderate stretch is perceived in the hamstring muscle group. This position is maintained for 30 seconds to 1 minute followed by a release of the stretch. The exercise is repeated as often as possible during the day with the minimum being six stretches, six times per day.

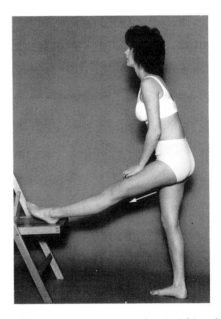

Fig. 11.4 Home exercise program for stretching the hamstring muscles.

iliac crest and the anterior superior iliac spine. The extensibility of the hamstring muscle group has been reached when the innominate bone is felt to flex (posteriorly rotate).

The patient is instructed to hold this position while the therapist attempts to further increase the femoral flexion at the hip joint. The contraction may be either isometric or eccentric and is held for up to five seconds followed by a period of complete relaxation. The femur is taken to the limit of the new physiological range of motion and the technique repeated from this point.

To specifically stretch the individual muscles of the hamstring muscle group, the starting position of the femur and the tibia may be altered in the following manner: biceps femoris—medially rotate/adduct the femur and medially rotate the tibia; semimembranosus/semitendinosus—laterally rotate/abduct the femur and laterally rotate the tibia.

Home exercise program (Fig. 11.4)

With the patient standing, the femur is flexed at the hip joint to the physiological limit of the

The exercise can be modified to specifically stretch the components of the hamstring muscle group by altering the starting position of the lower extremity. Medial rotation of the femur and tibia, combined with adduction of the femur prior to forward bending of the pelvic girdle, will maximally stretch the biceps femoris muscle. Lateral rotation of the femur and tibia, combined with abduction of the femur prior to forward bending of the pelvic girdle, will maximally stretch the semimembranosus and semitendinosus muscles.

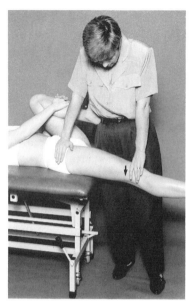

Fig. 11.5

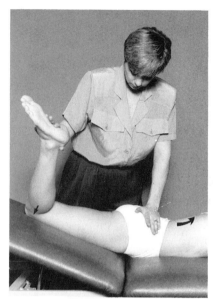

Fig. 11.6

Figs 11.5 and 11.6   Two active mobilization techniques for stretching the iliopsoas muscle.

Iliopsoas

Active mobilization (Fig. 11.5)

With the patient supine, lying at the end of the table, one femur is fully flexed against the trunk, held by the patient and supported against the therapist's lateral thorax. The anterior aspect of the iliac crest and the anterior superior iliac spine of the limb being stretched are palpated with the cranial hand. With the caudal hand, the therapist guides the femur into extension, with the knee extended, until the physiological length of the iliopsoas muscle has been reached.

The patient is instructed to hold this position while the therapist attempts to further increase the femoral extension at the hip joint. The contraction may be either isometric or eccentric and is held for up to five seconds followed by a period of complete relaxation. The femur is taken to the limit of the new physiological range of motion and the technique repeated from this point.

Maximal stretching of the iliopsoas muscle (Fig. 11.6) is achieved by having the patient lie prone with the vertebral column laterally flexed away from the muscle being stretched and the non-involved extremity supported on the floor such that the femur is flexed at the hip joint.[31] The involved extremity is then medially rotated at the hip joint with the knee flexed to 90° and supported in this position by the therapist. Femoral extension is achieved by elevating the end of the table. The active mobilization is performed by instructing the patient to flex the femur into the table, to hold the contraction for up to five seconds and then to completely relax. The femur is passively taken to the new physiological range of motion and the mobilization repeated.

Home exercise program (Fig. 11.7)

This muscle is very difficult to effectively stretch on one's own. The best method is to teach a relative the active mobilization procedure. Alternately, the following exercise can be given. With the patient standing, the non-involved extremity is flexed onto a stool or chair and the involved extremity extended and medially rotated behind the patient. From this position, the patient stretches forward, thus flexing the non-involved extremity and extending the involved extremity until moderate

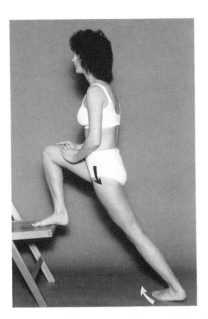

Fig. 11.7 Home exercise program for stretching the iliopsoas muscle.

stretch is perceived in the iliopsoas muscle. This position is maintained for 30 seconds to 1 minute followed by a release of the stretch. The exercise is repeated as often as possible during the day with the minimum being six stretches, six times per day.

Rectus femoris

Active mobilization (Fig. 11.8)

With the patient supine, lying at the end of the table, one femur is fully flexed against the trunk, held by the patient and supported against the therapist's lateral thorax. The anterior aspect of the iliac crest and the anterior superior iliac spine of the limb being stretched are palpated with the cranial hand. With the caudal hand, the therapist guides the femur into extension, with the knee flexed, until the physiological length of the rectus femoris muscle has been reached.

The patient is instructed to hold this position while the therapist attempts to flex the knee further. The contraction may be either isometric or eccentric and is held for up to five seconds followed by a period of complete relaxation. The tibia is taken to the limit of the new physiological range of motion and the technique repeated from this point.

Maximal stretching of the rectus femoris muscle (Fig. 11.9) is achieved by having the patient lie prone with the non-involved extremity supported on the floor such that the femur is flexed at the hip joint.[31] The involved extremity is then flexed at the knee joint to

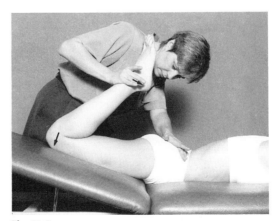

Fig. 11.8   **Fig. 11.9**

Figs 11.8 and 11.9 Two active mobilization techniques for stretching the rectus femoris muscle.

the physiological limit and supported in this position by the therapist. Further stretch is achieved by extending the femur at the hip joint by elevating the end of the table. The active mobilization is performed by instructing the patient to flex the femur into the table and to extend the tibia against the therapist's resistance. The contraction is held for up to five seconds followed by a period of complete relaxation. The tibia and the femur are passively taken to the new physiological range of motion and the mobilization repeated.

Home exercise program (Fig. 11.10)

With the patient standing, the femur is initially flexed at the hip joint and the tibia flexed at the knee joint. The ankle is grasped just proximal to the talocrural joint and the knee flexion maintained while the femur is passively extended at the hip joint until moderate stretch is perceived in the rectus femoris muscle. This position is maintained for 30 seconds to 1 minute followed by a release of the stretch. The exercise is repeated as often as possible during the day with the minimum being six stretches, six times per day.

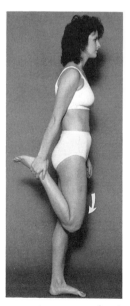

Fig. 11.10 Home exercise program for stretching the rectus femoris muscle.

Tensor fascia lata

Active mobilization[31]

To actively mobilize the right tensor fascia lata muscle, the patient is positioned in right side-lying with the left hip and knee comfortably flexed. The anterolateral aspect of the right femur is grasped with the caudal hand and the flexed right knee supported by the therapist's caudal hand and forearm. The cranial hand stabilizes the posterior aspect of the pelvic girdle. The femur is taken to the physiological limit of the tensor fascia lata muscle by passively extending, adducting and laterally rotating the femur at the hip joint.

At this position, the patient is instructed to resist further extension, adduction and lateral rotation of the femur. The contraction may be either isometric or eccentric and is held for up to five seconds followed by a period of complete relaxation. The femur is taken to the limit of the new physiological range of motion and the technique repeated from this point.

Home exercise program[91] *(Fig. 11.11)*

To passively stretch the right tensor fascia lata muscle, the patient is instructed to stand with the left leg crossed over the right. The patient

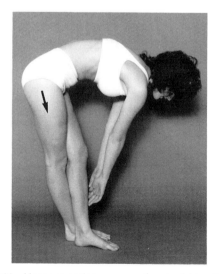

Fig. 11.11 Home exercise program for stretching the right tensor fascia lata muscle.

is instructed to forward bend from this position while reaching towards the medial side of the right ankle with the right hand. This motion induces lateral rotation/adduction of the flexed pelvic girdle on the femur, thus stretching the right tensor fascia lata muscle. This position is maintained for 30 seconds to 1 minute followed by a release of the stretch. The exercise is repeated as often as possible during the day with the minimum being six stretches, six times per day.

Adductors

Active mobilization (Fig. 11.12)

With the patient supine, lying at the end of the table, one femur is fully flexed against the trunk, held by the patient and supported against the therapist's lateral thorax. The anterior aspect of the iliac crest and the anterior superior iliac spine of the limb being stretched are palpated with the cranial hand. With the caudal hand, the therapist guides the femur into abduction until the physiological limit of the adductor muscles has been reached. The degree of femoral flexion/

extension, medial/lateral rotation can be varied according to the pattern of restriction found.

The patient is instructed to resist further abduction from this position. The contraction may be either isometric or eccentric and is held for up to five seconds followed by a period of complete relaxation. The femur is taken to the limit of the new physiological range of motion and the technique repeated from this point.

Home exercise program (Fig. 11.13)

With the patient standing, the femur is abducted at the hip joint to the physiological limit of the adductor muscle group while maintaining the vertebral column in a neutral position and the knee joint in full extension. From this position, the patient flexes the supporting extremity, thus inducing further abduction of the contralateral limb until moderate stretch is perceived in the tight adductor muscle group. This position is maintained for 30 seconds to 1 minute followed by a release of the stretch. The exercise is repeated as often as possible during the day

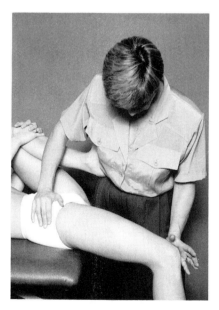

Fig. 11.12 Active mobilization technique for stretching the adductor muscles.

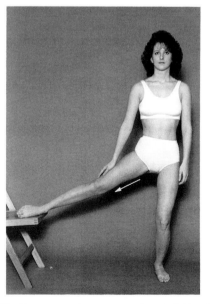

Fig. 11.13 Home exercise program for stretching the adductor muscles.

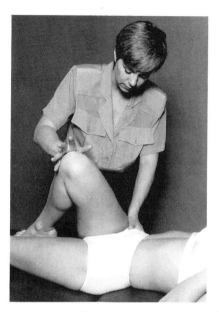

Fig. 11.14 Active mobilization technique for stretching the piriformis muscle.

with the minimum being six stretches, six times per day.

Piriformis

Active mobilization (Fig. 11.14)

With the patient lying supine, the lower extremity is grasped at the flexed knee. The lateral aspect of the iliac crest and the anterior superior iliac spine are palpated with the cranial hand while the caudal hand flexes the femur to 60° of flexion. At this point, the piriformis muscle acts as a pure abductor of the femur. Before 60° it also laterally rotates the femur, while after 60° it medially rotates the femur. From 60° of femoral flexion, the femur is guided into adduction with the caudal hand while the cranial hand monitors the subsequent medial rotation (inflaring) of the innominate bone. The extensibility of the piriformis muscle has been reached when the innominate bone is felt to medially rotate, and although further adduction of the femur is possible, it is secondary to the medial rotation of the innominate bone. If the femur is taken beyond 60° of flexion, lateral femoral rotation is also required to fully stretch the muscle.

The patient is instructed to resist further adduction from this position (if the femur is flexed to 60°), to resist adduction/lateral rotation (if the femur is flexed beyond 60°), and adduction/medial rotation (if the femur is flexed less than 60°). The contraction may be either isometric or eccentric and is held for up to five seconds followed by a period of complete relaxation. The femur is taken to the limit of the new physiological range of motion and the technique repeated from this point.

Home exercise program (Fig. 11.15)

With the patient lying supine, the lower extremity is grasped at the flexed knee with one hand and at the ankle with the other. The femur is flexed/adducted and laterally rotated to the physiological limit of the piriformis muscle until moderate stretch is perceived in the buttock. This position is maintained for 30 seconds to 1 minute followed by a release of the stretch. The exercise is repeated as often as possible during the day with the minimum being six stretches, six times per day.

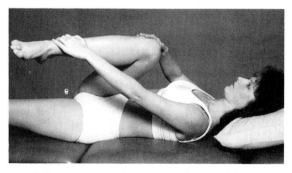

Fig. 11.15 Home exercise program for stretching the piriformis muscle.

PHASIC MUSCLES

Relative to the pelvic girdle, the phasic muscles which tend to weaken include the:
1. abdominals
2. gluteus maximus, medius, minimus
3. vastus lateralis, intermedius and medialis.
Clinically, the weakened phasic muscles reduce the dynamic stability of the pelvic

girdle, thus predisposing the individual to recurrent articular strains of the lumbosacral junction as well as the sacroiliac joint.

The treatment includes a progressive exercise program designed to strengthen the weakened muscle group, combined with ergonomic retraining (which is discussed later.)

Abdominals

Preliminary exercises (Fig. 11.16)

With the patient lying supine, the hips and knees are comfortably flexed. The patient is instructed to flatten the lumbar spine into the table, thus inducing a pelvic tilt. Careful observation is necessary when teaching this exercise since many patients will attempt to flatten the spine by pushing with their feet rather than using the abdominal muscle group. The position is maintained for up to 10 seconds followed by a brief rest period. The number of repetitions is progressively increased.

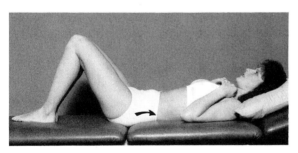

Fig. 11.16 A preliminary exercise for strengthening the abdominals.

The exercise is progressed when a pelvic tilt is successfully achieved using the abdominal muscles. While maintaining the pelvic tilt position, the patient is instructed to straighten one extremity to 45° of femoral flexion. The position is maintained for up to 10 seconds followed by a brief rest period. The number of repetitions is progressively increased. *If the patient is able to maintain the pelvic tilt*, the exercise can be progressed.

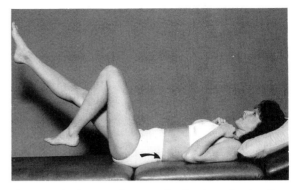

Fig. 11.17 An intermediary exercise for strengthening the abdominals.

Intermediary exercises (Fig. 11.17)

With the patient lying supine, the hips and knees are comfortably flexed. The patient is instructed to induce a pelvic tilt and to maintain this position while straightening one extremity to 45° followed by lifting the opposite foot off of the table (but not extending it as yet). The position is maintained for up to 10 seconds followed by a brief rest period. The number of repetitions is progressively increased.

If the patient is able to maintain the pelvic tilt, the exercise can be progressed to straightening both lower extremities to 45°. The position is maintained for up to 10 seconds followed by a brief rest period. The number of repetitions is progressively increased.

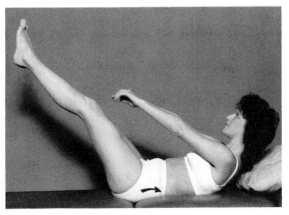

Fig. 11.18 An advanced exercise for strengthening the abdominals.

138 / *The Pelvic Girdle*

Advanced exercises (Fig. 11.18)

With the patient lying supine, the hips and knees are comfortable flexed. The patient is instructed to induce a pelvic tilt and to maintain this position while straightening both lower extremities to 45°. While maintaining this position, the head and shoulders are slightly lifted off of the table, first in the sagittal body plane and then in the oblique body planes. The position is maintained for up to 10 seconds followed by a brief rest period. The number of repetitions is progressively increased.

Gluteus maximus, medius, minimus
Vastus lateralis, intermedius, medialis

These muscles can be strengthened individually via specific exercise programs which need not be described here. The functional approach to rehabilitating these muscles involves weight-bearing exercises which integrate the neuromuscular function of the lumbo-pelvic-hip complex. These exercises can then be integrated into the ergonomic retraining program.

With the patient standing, the feet are spread hip-width distance apart and approximately 12 inches (30.5 cm) away from a wall. In this position, the patient is instructed to flex the pelvic girdle (i.e. pelvic tilt), thus flattening the lumbar spine, and to semi-flex the hips and knees. This position is maintained for up to 45 seconds followed by a brief rest period. The number of repetitions is progressively increased.

The exercise is progressed by instructing the patient to shift the body weight from one extremity to the other in the coronal body plane while maintaining the vertebral column in an erect position (i.e. no lateral bending) (Fig. 11.19). The patient is thus taught to use the lower extremities, as opposed to the lumbar spine, to transfer the body weight in a coronal plane. The ability to dissociate motion of the lower extremities from the vertebral column is critical to the successful rehabilitation of the lumbo-pelvic-hip complex.

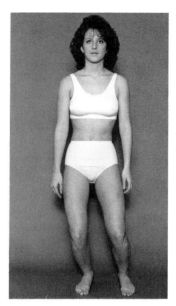

Fig. 11.19 A home exercise for strengthening the hip and knee extensors as well as for re-educating the optimal transference of the body weight in the coronal plane by using the lower extremities and not the vertebral column.

This exercise also happens to strengthen both the glutei and the quadriceps muscle groups.

POSTURAL AND ERGONOMIC RETRAINING

Sitting

The ideal sitting position (Fig. 11.20) is the one which maintains the spine in a neutral position, thus preserving the natural cervical, thoracic and lumbar curves, as well as directing the line of gravity through the lumbosacral junction along the arcuate lines of the innominate bones through to the massive ischial tuberosities. If the body weight is allowed to pass anterior or posterior to this ideal position (Figs 11.21, 11.22), excessive static stresses will be induced through the lumbo-pelvic-hip complex, thus facilitating breakdown of the tissues.

The average chair appears to be designed for the 5 ft 10 in (178 cm) man. Individuals less than this height must slide forward in the chair if the feet are to reach the ground. This motion places the line of gravity behind the

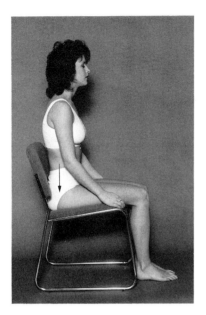

Fig. 11.20 The optimal sitting posture preserves the natural cervical, thoracic and lumbar curves.

ischial tuberosities, thus encouraging flexion of the lumbar vertebral column and the pelvic girdle (i.e. slouching). Individuals greater than this height have more difficulty controlling the optimal posture of the upper quadrant. To reach a desk top, they must lower the trunk, thereby flexing the cervicothoracic and thoracic portions of the vertebral column.

Adjusting the work height, as well as the visual field, is critical to successfully maintaining an optimal sitting posture. If the desk is too high, the shoulder girdle must be elevated to write, which can induce a lateral bend of the vertebral column. If the desk is too low, the shoulder girdle must descend, thus encouraging flexion of the vertebral column. Careful revision of the patient's sitting posture is required if the patient's occupation and/or leisure activity requires the habitual use of this position.

The goal is to position the lumbo-pelvic-hip complex in the optimal posture of balance such that the osseous components of the unit bear the majority of the stresses (see Ch. 5).

Erect standing

It has been shown[7] that among the mammals man has the most efficient posture in bipedal stance. In the lumbo-pelvic-hip region, intermittent bursts of activity from the gluteus medius, tensor fascia lata and hamstring muscles are required to control postural sway. Constant activity has been reported[7] in the

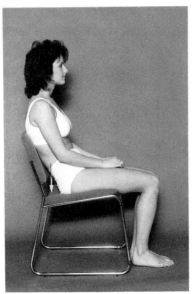

Fig. 11.21

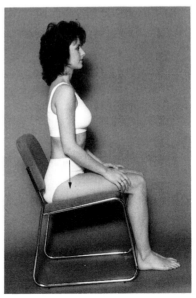

Fig. 11.22

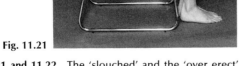

Figs 11.21 and 11.22 The 'slouched' and the 'over erect' sitting postures.

iliopsoas muscle to support the iliofemoral ligament of the hip joint, as well as in the internal oblique muscle to protect the inguinal canal. All other muscle groups are quiescent when bipedal posture is optimal. Deviation from this economical position results in the immediate recruitment of both the trunk and femoral musculature, thus dramatically increasing the energy expenditure of standing still.

Where is this optimal position? To review, if the body is viewed from the lateral aspect, a vertical line should pass through the following points (see Fig. 7.1):

1. the external auditory meatus
2. the bodies of the cervical vertebrae
3. the glenohumeral joint
4. slightly anterior to the bodies of the thoracic vertebrae transecting the vertebrae at the thoracolumbar junction
5. the bodies of the lumbar vertebrae
6. the sacral promontory
7. slightly posterior to the coronal axis of the hip joint
8. slightly anterior to the coronal axis of the knee joint
9. slightly anterior to the talocrural joint
10. the naviculo-calcaneo-cuboid joint.

Fortunately, we are rarely required to stand perfectly still; however, some tasks, such as ironing, do require prolonged periods of relative immobility of the lower quadrant. If the position of optimal postural balance is lost, the energy expenditure required to stand still will increase. Excessive static stresses will then be placed on the tissues of the lumbo-pelvic-hip complex, facilitating their breakdown.

Frequently altering the standing posture is one means of coping with relative immobility. The unilateral elevation of one foot onto a low stool should not be habitually encouraged unless alternated with the opposite extremity. Ideally, the patient should be taught how to achieve the optimal posture of the lumbo-pelvic-hip complex as well as encouraged to frequently move both into and out of this position.

Lifting

The biomechanics of the optimal lifting technique have been described in Chapter 5. If the myofascial function of the lumbo-pelvic-hip complex has been restored (see the beginning of this chapter), the patient should be able to learn to lift ideally. The key points to teach include:

1. The shoulder girdle *must* stay in the same coronal plane as the pelvic girdle for the entire duration of the lift. This requires the maintenance of the pelvic tilt position (i.e. strong abdominals and hip extensors).
2. The load must never move outside of the pedal base (i.e. keep the load close to the body). This requires strong quadriceps and hip abductor muscles. When transferring patients up/down the bed, the magnitude of the transfer must be confined to the coronal dimensions of the pedal base. If this point is neglected, the shoulder girdle will have had to move away from the coronal plane of the pelvic girdle, thus necessitating the loss of the pelvic tilt.
3. The load must be tested prior to being lifted and its weight never assumed. Obviously, if the load is too heavy, help is required.

In summary, optimal and therefore safe loading and unloading of the lumbo-pelvic-hip region during activities of daily living can occur when the myokinematics and the myokinetics subserve the kinetic and kinematic requirements of the bones and joints they stabilize and move. The co-ordinated muscle response is dependent upon complex peripheral and central feedback mechanisms which integrate the osseous, articular and muscular function. Successful rehabilitation requires attention to all these aspects of the lumbo-pelvic-hip complex.

References

1 Abergel R P 1984 Biostimulation of procollagen production by low energy lasers in human skin fibroblast cultures. Journal of Investigative Dermatology 82: 395

2 Adams J C 1973 Outline of orthopaedics, 7th edn. Churchill, London

3 Aitken G S 1986 Syndromes of lumbo-pelvic dysfunction. In: Grieve G P (ed) Modern manual therapy of the vertebral column. Churchill Livingstone, Edinburgh, Ch 43, p 473

4 Albee F H 1909 A study of the anatomy and the clinical importance of the sacroiliac joint. Journal of the American Medical Association 53: 1273

5 Anderson C K, Herberts T N, Ortengren R 1977 Quantitative electromyographic studies of back muscle activity related to posture and loading. Orthopedic Clinics of North America 8: 85

6 Astrom J 1975 Pre-operative effect of fenestration upon intraosseous pressures in patients with osteoarthrosis of the hip. Acta Orthopaedica Scandinavcia 46: 963

7 Basmajian J V, Deluca C J 1985 Muscles alive their functions revealed by electromyography. Williams & Wilkins, Baltimore

8 Bassett C A L 1968 Biologic significance of piezoelectricity. Calcified Tissue Research 1: 252

9 Beal M C 1982 The sacroiliac problem: review of anatomy, mechanics, and diagnosis. Journal of the American Osteopathic Association 81: 667

10 Bellamy N, Park W, Rooney P J 1983 What do we know about the sacroiliac joint? Seminars in Arthritis and Rheumatism 12: 282

11 Bogduk N 1980 A reappraisal of the anatomy of the human lumbar erector spinae. Journal of Anatomy 131: 525

12 Bogduk N 1983 The innervation of the lumbar spine. Spine 8: 286

13 Bogduk N 1984 The menisci of the lumbar zygapophysial joints: a review of their anatomy and clinical significance. Spine 9: 454

14 Bogduk N 1985 Low back pain. Australian Family Physician 14: 1168

15 Bogduk N 1986 The anatomy and function of the lumbar back muscles. In: Grieve G P (ed) Modern manual therapy of the vertebral column. Churchill Livingstone, Edinburgh, Ch 13, p 138

16 Bogduk N, Twomey L T 1987 Clinical anatomy of the lumbar spine. Churchill Livingstone, Melbourne

17 Bowen V, Cassidy J D 1981 Macroscopic and microscopic anatomy of the sacroiliac joint from embryonic life until the eighth decade. Spine 6: 620

18 Bradlay K C 1985 The posterior primary rami of segmental nerves. In: Glasgow E F, Twomey, L T, Scull E R, Kleynhans A M (eds) Aspects of manipulative therapy, 2nd edn. Churchill Livingstone, Melbourne, Ch 9, p 59

19 Brooke R 1930 The pelvic joints during and after parturition and pregnancy. The Practitioner, London, p 307

20 Brooke R 1924 The sacro-iliac joint. Journal of Anatomy 58: 299

21 Chamberlain W E 1930 The symphysis pubis in the roentgen examination of the sacroiliac joint. American Journal of Roentgenology 24: 621

22 Colachis S C, Worden R E, Bechtol C O, Strohm B R 1963 Movement of the sacroiliac joint in the adult male: a preliminary report. Archives of Physical Medicine and Rehabilitation 44: 490

23 Crock H V 1980 An atlas of the arterial supply of the head and neck of the femur in man. Clinical Orthopaedics and Related Research 152: 17

24 Cyriax J 1954 Textbook of orthopaedic medicine. Cassell, London

25 de Diemerbroeck I 1689 The anatomy of human bodies. Translated by W Salmon Brewster, London

26 Dee R 1969 Structure and function of hip joint innervation. Annals of the Royal College of Surgeons of England 45: 357

27 Dvorak J, Dvorak V 1984 Manual medicine diagnostics. Thieme-Stratton, New York

28 Egund N, Olsson T H, Schmid H 1978 Movements in the sacro-iliac joints demonstrated with roentgen stereophotogrammetry. Acta Radiologica 19: 833

29 Encyclopedia Britannica 1981 15th edn, Vol 7. William Benter, Chicago

30 Evjenth O, Hamberg J 1984 Muscle stretching in manual therapy, a clinical manual; the spinal column and the TM—joint. Alfta Rehab Forlag, Sweden

31 Evjenth O, Hamberg J 1984 Muscle stretching in manual therapy, a clinical manual; the extremities. Alfta Rehab Forlag, Sweden

32 Farfan H F 1973 Mechanical disorders of the low back. Lea & Febiger, Philadelphia

33 Farfan H F 1975 Muscular mechanism of the lumbar spine and the position of power and efficiency. Orthopedic Clinics of North America 8: 199

34 Farfan H F 1978 The biomechanical advantage of lordosis and hip extension for upright activity. Spine 3: 336

35 Fothergill W E 1896 Walcher's position in parturition. British Medical Journal 2: 1292

36 Fowler C 1984 The upslip. Proceedings of the International Federation of Orthopaedic Manipulative Therapists—5th, Vancouver, p 122

37 Fowler C 1986 Muscle energy techniques for pelvic dysfunction. In: Grieve G P (ed) Modern manual therapy of the vertebral column. Churchill Livingstone, Edinburgh, Ch 77, p 805

38 Fryette H H 1914 Four innominate lesions—their cause, diagnosis and treatment. Journal of American Osteopathic Association 14: 3

39 Fryette H H 1954 Principles of osteopathic technique. American Academy of Osteopathy, Colorado

40 Gilmore K L 1986 Biomechanics of the lumbar motion segment. In: Grieve G P (ed) Modern manual therapy of the vertebral column. Churchill Livingstone, Edinburgh, Ch 9, p 103

41 Gilraine F, Nihls, M 1985 A sacroiliac support for use during pregnancy. Canadian Orthopaedic Manipulative Therapists Proceedings, British Columbia, p 23

42 Goldthwait J E, Osgood R B 1905 A consideration of the pelvic articulations from an anatomical, pathological andd clinical standpoint. Boston Medical and Surgical Journal 152: 593

43 Goodall J 1979 Life and death at Gombe. National Geographic 155(5): 592

44 Gracovetsky S, Farfan H F 1986 The optimum spine. Spine 11: 543

45 Gracovetsky S, Farfan H F, Lamy C 1981 The mechanism of the lumbar spine. Spine 6: 249

46 Gracovetsky S, Farfan H, Helluer C 1985 The abdominal mechanism. Spine 10: 317

47 Gregersen G, Lucas D B 1967 An in vivo study of axial rotation of the human thoraco-lumbar spine. Journal of Bone and Joint Surgery 49A: 247

48 Grieve G P 1981 Common vertebral joint problems. Churchill Livingstone, Edinburgh

49 Grieve G P 1983 The hip. Physiotherapy 69: 196

50 Grieve G P (ed) 1986 Modern manual therapy of the vertebral column. Churchill Livingstone, Edinburgh

51 Grieve G P 1986 Lumbar instability. In: Grieve G P (ed) Modern manual therapy of the vertebral column. Churchill Livingstone, Edinburgh, Ch 40, p 416

52 Hagen R 1974 Pelvic girdle relaxation from an orthopaedic point of view. Acta Orthopaedica Scandinavica 45: 550

53 Harris N H, Murray R O 1974 Lesions of the symphysis in athletes. British Medical Journal 4: 211

54 Hutter M J An anatomical review of the hip. Bulletin of the Orthopaedic Section of the American Physical Therapy Association 2: 5

55 Inman V T, Ralston H J, Todd F 1981 Human walking. Williams & Wilkins, Baltimore

56 Janda V 1986 Muscle weakness and inhibition (pseudoparesis) in back pain syndromes. In: Grieve G P (ed) Modern manual therapy of the vertebral column. Churchill Livingstone, Edinburgh, Ch 19, p 197

57 Janda V 1978 Muscles, central nervous motor regulation and back problems. In: Korr I (ed) The neurobiologic mechanisms in manipulative therapy. Plenum Press, London, p 27

58 Janda V 1976 The muscular factor in the pathogenesis of back pain syndrome. Physiotherapy Symposium, Oslo

59 Jarcho J 1929 Value of Walcher position in contracted pelvis with special reference to its effect on true conjugate diameter. Surgery, Gynecology and Obstetrics 49: 854

60 Kapandji I A 1970 The physiology of the joints II: the lower limb, 2nd edn. Churchill Livingstone, Edinburgh

61 Kapandji I A 1974 The physiology of joints III: the trunk and vertebral column, 2nd edn. Churchill Livingstone, Edinburgh

62 Kappel D A, Zilber S, Ketchum L D 1973 In vivo electrophysiology of tendons and applied current during tendon healing. In: Llaurado J G, Battocletti J H (eds) Biologic and clinical effects of low-frequency magnetic and electric fields. C C Thomas, Illinois, Ch 21, p 252

63 Kappler R E 1982 Postural balance and motion patterns. Journal of the American Osteopathic Association 81(9): 598

64 Keagy R D, Brumlik J 1966 Direct electromyography of the psoas major muscle in man. Journal of Bone and Joint Surgery 48A: 1377

65 Kirkaldy-Willis W H (ed) 1983 Managing low back pain. Churchill Livingstone, New York

66 Kirkaldy-Willis W H, Hill R J 1979 A more precise diagnosis for low back pain. Spine 4: 102

67 Kirkaldy-Willis W H, Wedge J H, Yong-Hing K, Reilly J 1978 Pathology and pathogenesis of lumbar spondylosis and stenosis. Spine 3: 319

68 Lawson T L, Foley W D, Carrera G F, Berland L L 1982 The sacroiliac joints: anatomic, plain roentgenographic, and computed tomographic analysis. Journal of Computer Assisted Tomography 6(2): 307

69 Lee D 1986 Principles and practice of muscle energy and functional techniques. In: Grieve G P (ed) Modern manual therapy of the vertebral column. Churchill Livingstone, Edinburgh, Ch 59, p 640

70 Lee D G, Walsh M C 1985 Bones in space. Proceedings of the Canadian Orthopaedic Manipulative Therapists, British Columbia, p 39

71 Lee D G, Walsh M C 1986 A workbook of manual therapy techniques for the vertebral column and pelvic girdle. Nascent, Delta

72 Lovett R W 1903 A contribution to the study of the mechanics of the spine. American Journal of Anatomy 2: 457

73 Luk K D K, Ho H C, Leong J C Y 1986 The iliolumbar ligament: a study of its anatomy, development and clinical significance. Journal of Bone and Joint Surgery 68B: 197

74 Lumsden R M, Morris J M 1968 An in vivo study of axial rotation and immobilization of the lumbosacral joint. Journal of Bone and Joint Surgery 50A: 1591

75 Lynch F W 1920 The pelvic articulations during pregnancy, labor, and the puerperium. Surgery, Gynecology and Obstetrics 30: 575

76 MacConaill M A, Basmajian J V 1977 Muscles and movements; a basis for human kinesiology, 2nd edn. Krieger, New York

77 MacDonald G R, Hunt T E 1951 Sacro-iliac joints observations on the gross and histological changes in the various age groups. Canadian Medical Association Journal 66: 157

78 Macnab I 1977 Backache. Williams & Wilkins, Baltimore

79 McQueen P M 1977 The piriformis syndrome. Physiotherapy Society Manipulation Newsletter, Melbourne 8: 1

80 Maxwell T D 1978 The piriformis muscle and its relation to the long-legged syndrome. Journal of the Canadian Chiropractic Association July: 51

81 Meadows J 1985 Pelvic arthrokinematics. Proceedings of the International Federation of Orthopaedic Manipulative therapists—5th, Vancouver, p 96

82 Meckel J F 1832 Manual of general descriptive and pathologic anatomy. Philadelphia

83 Meisenbach R O 1911 Sacro-iliac relaxation; with analysis of eighty-four cases. Surgery, Gynecology and Obstetrics 12: 411

84 Melzak R, Wall P D 1965 Pain mechanisms: a new theory. Science 150: 971

85 Mennell J B 1952 The science and art of joint manipulation. Churchill, London

86 Mester E 1971 Effects of laser rays on wound healing. The American Journal of Surgery 122: 532

87 Meyer G H 1878 Der Mechanismus der Symphysis sacroiliaca. Archiv fur Anatomie und Physiologie 1: 1

88 Mitchell F 1965 Structural pelvic function. Year Book: Academy of Applied Osteopathy. Carmel, California

89 Mitchell F L, Moran P S, Pruzzo N A 1979 An evaluation and treatment manual of osteopathic muscle energy procedures. Mitchell, Moran and Pruzzo, Mo

90 Mixter W J, Barr J S 1934 Rupture of intervertebral disc with involvement of the spinal cord. New England Journal of Medicine 211: 210

91 Mortensen-Young S 1987 Personal communication

92 Nelson H, Jurmain R 1985 Introduction to physical anthropology, 3rd edn. West Publishing, St Paul

93 Pace J B, Nagle D 1976 The piriformis syndrome. Western Journal of Medicine 124: 435

94 Peacock E E 1984 Wound repair, 3rd edn. W B Saunders, London

95 Pearcy M, Portek I, Shepherd J 1984 Three-dimensional X-ray analysis of normal movement in the lumbar spine. Spine 9: 294

96 Pearcy M, Tibrewal S B 1984 Axial rotation and lateral bending in the normal lumbar spine measured by three-dimensional radiography. Spine 9: 582

97 Pettman E A, Meadows J 1986 Personal communication

98 Pitkin H C, Pheasant H C 1936 Sacroarthrogenetic telalagia II. A study of sacral mobility. Journal of Bone and Joint Surgery 18: 365

99 Pratt W A 1952 The lumbopelvic torsion syndrome. Journal of the American Osteopathic Association 51: 97

100 Reilly J, Yong-Hing K, Mackay R W, Kirkaldy-Willis W H 1978 Pathological anatomy of the lumbar spine. In: Helfet A J, Gruebel-Lee D M (eds) Disorders of the lumbar spine. J B Lippincott, Philadelphia

101 Resnick D, Niwayama G, Goergen T G 1975 Degenerative disease of the sacroiliac joint. Journal of Investigative Radiology 10: 608

102 Reynolds H M 1980 Three-dimensional kinematics in the pelvic girdle. Journal of the American Osteopathic Association 80: 277

103 Rodman P S, McHenry M 1980 Bioenergetics and the origin of hominid bipedalism. American Journal of Physical Anthropology 52: 103

104 Romer A S 1959 A shorter version of the vertebrate body. W B Saunders, Philadelphia

105 Rothman R H, Simeone F A 1975 Spine, Vol. IV. W B Saunders, London

106 Sashin D 1930 A critical analysis of the anatomy and the pathologic changes of the sacro-iliac joints. Journal of Bone and Joint Surgery 12: 891

107 Schunke G B 1938 The anatomy and development of the sacro-iliac joint in man. The Anatomical Record 72: 313

108 Siffert R S, Feldman D J 1980 The growing hip. Acta Orthopaedica Belgica 46: 443

109 Singleton M C, LeVeau B F 1975 The hip joint: structure, stability, and stress. Physical Therapy 55: 957

110 Solonen K A 1957 The sacro-iliac joint in the light of anatomical roentgenological and clinical studies. Acta Orthopaedica Scandinavica Supplement 26

111 Stein P L, Rowe B M 1982 Physical anthropology, 3rd edn. McGraw–Hill, New York

112 Stokes I A F 1986 Three-dimensional biplanar radiography of the lumbar spine. In: Grieve G P (ed) Modern manual therapy of the vertebral column. Churchill Livingstone, Edinburgh, Ch 54, p 576

113 Strachan W F, Beckwith C G, Larson N J 1938 A study of the mechanics of the sacroiliac joint. Journal of the American Osteopathic Association 37: 576

114 Strayer L M 1971 Embryology of the human hip joint. Clinical Orthopaedics 74: 221

115 Sunderland S 1978 Traumatised nerves, roots and ganglia: musculo-skeletal factors and neuropathological consequences. In: Korr (ed) The neurobiologic mechanisms in manipulative therapy. Plenum Press, London, p 137

116 Sweeting R 1984 Hypermobility of the sacroiliac joint. Proceedings of the International Federation of Manipulative Therapists—5th, Vancouver, p 258

117 Swindler D R, Wood C D 1982 An atlas of primate gross anatomy baboon, chimpanzee, and man. Robert E. Krieger, Florida

118 Tait G B, Dee R, Wyke B D 1969 Reflex function of the ligamentum capitus femoris. Annals of the Rheumatic Diseases 28: 554

119 Travell J G, Rinzler S H 1952 The myofascial genesis of pain. Postgraduate Medicine 11: 425

120 Trotter M 1937 Accessory sacro-iliac articulations. American Journal of Physical Anthropology 22: 247

121 Troup J D G 1977 Dynamic factors in the analysis of stoop and crouch lifting methods: a methodological approach to the development of safe materials handling standards. Orthopedic Clinics of North America 8: 201

122 Tuttle R H (ed) 1975 Primate functional morphology. Mouton, The Hague

123 Twomey L T, Taylor J R 1985 A quantitative study of the role of the posterior vertebral elements in sagittal movements of the lumbar vertebral column. In: Glasgow E F, Twomey L T, Scull E R, Kleynhans A M (eds) Aspects of manipulative therapy, 2nd edn. Churchill Livingstone, Melbourne, Ch 4, p 34

124 Twomey L T, Taylor J R 1986 The effects of ageing on the lumbar intervertebral discs. In: Grieve G P (ed) Modern manual therapy of the vertebral column. Churchill Livingstone, Edinburgh, Ch 12, p 129

125 Walker J M 1980 Morphological variants in the human fetal hip joint. Journal of Bone and Joint Surgery 62A: 1073

126 Walker J M 1980 Growth characteristics of the fetal ligament of the head of femur: significance in congenital hip disease. Yale Journal of Biology and Medicine 53: 307

127 Walker J M 1981 Histological study of the fetal development of the human acetabulum and labrum: significance in congenital hip disease. Yale Journal of Biology and Medicine 54: 255

128 Walker J M 1984 Age changes in the sacroiliac joint. Proceedings of the International Federation of Orthopaedic Manipulative Therapists—5th, Vancouver, p 250

129 Walker J M 1986 Age-related differences in the human sacroiliac joint: a histological study; implications for therapy. Journal of Orthopaedic and Sports Physical Therapy 7: 325

130 Walsh M C, Fowler C, Treloar D 1987 Personal communication

131 Warwick R, Williams P (eds) 1973 Gray's anatomy, 35th edn. Longman, London

132 Watanabe R S 1974 Embryology of the human hip. Clinical Orthopaedics 98: 8

133 Webster D F, Harvey W, Dyson M, Pond J B 1980 The role of ultrasound-induced cavitation in the 'in vitro' stimulation of collagen synthesis in human fibroblasts. Ultrasonic 18: 33

134 Weisl H 1954 The articular surfaces of the sacro-iliac joint and their relation to the movements of the sacrum. Acta Anatomica 22: 1

135 Weisl H 1955 The movements of the sacro-iliac joint. Acta Anatomica 23: 80

136 Wells P E 1986 The examination of the pelvic joints. In: Grieve G P (ed) Modern manual therapy of the vertebral column. Churchill Livingstone, Edinburgh, Ch 56, p 590

137 White A A, Panjabi M M 1978 The basic kinematics of the human spine. Spine 3: 12

138 Wilder D G, Pope M H, Frymoyer J W 1980 The functional topography of the sacroiliac joint. Spine 5: 575

139 Wroblewski B M 1978 Pain in osteoarthrosis of the hip. Practitioner 1315: 140

140 Wyke B D 1981 The neurology of joints: a review of general principles. Clinics in Rheumatic Diseases 7: 223

141 Wyke B D 1985 Articular neurology and manipulative therapy. In: Glasgow E F, Twomey L T, Scull E R, Kleynhans A M (eds) Aspects of manipulative therapy, 2nd edn. Churchill Livingstone, Melbourne, Ch 11, p 72

142 Young J 1940 Relaxation of the pelvic joints in pregnancy: pelvic arthropathy of pregnancy. Journal of Obstetrics and Gynecology 47: 493

143 Young J Z 1981 The life of vertebrates, 3rd edn. Clarenden Press, Oxford

Index